Assistive and Rehabilitation Engineering

Edited by Yves Rybarczyk

Published in London, United Kingdom

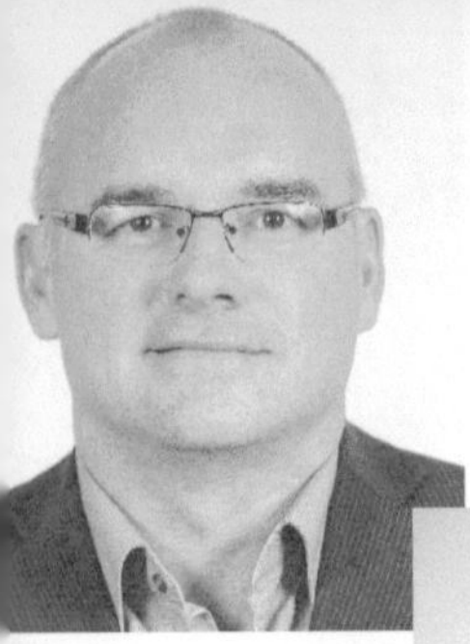
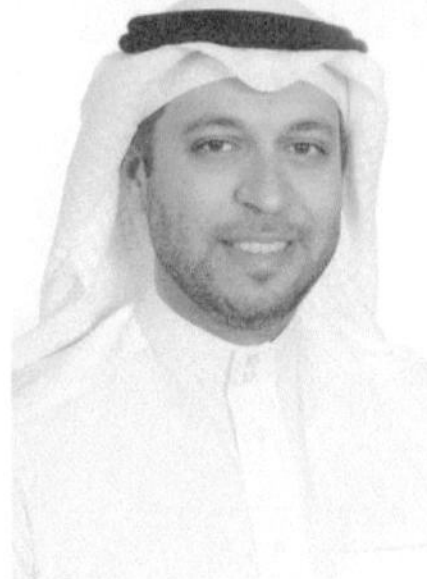
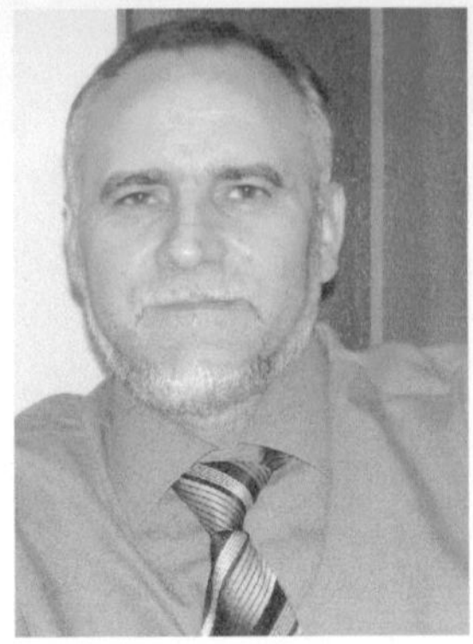
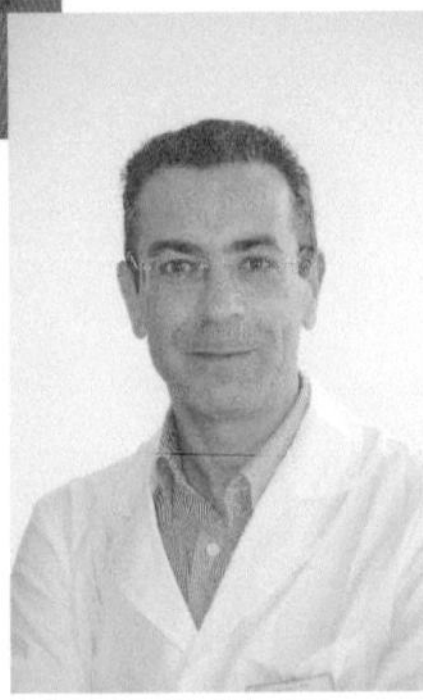
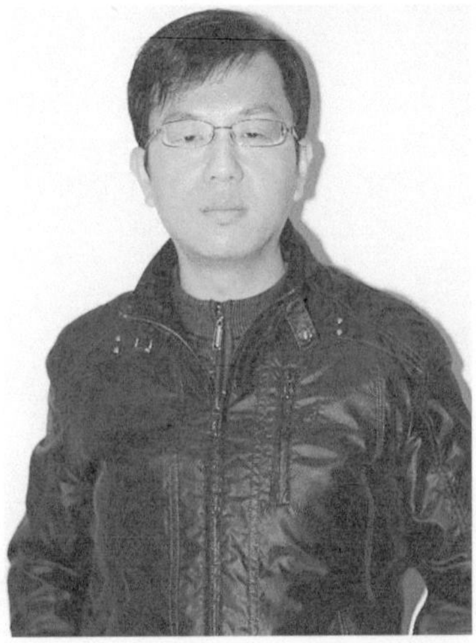
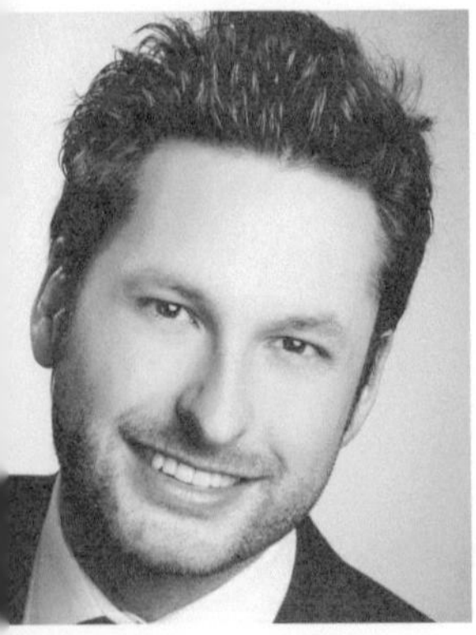
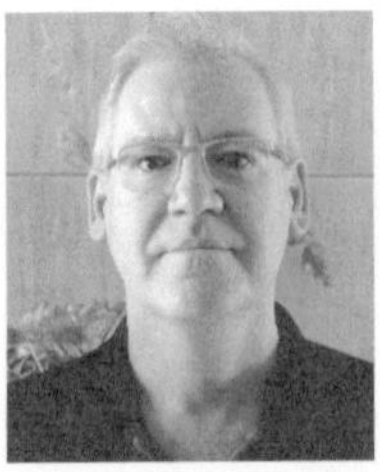

IntechOpen

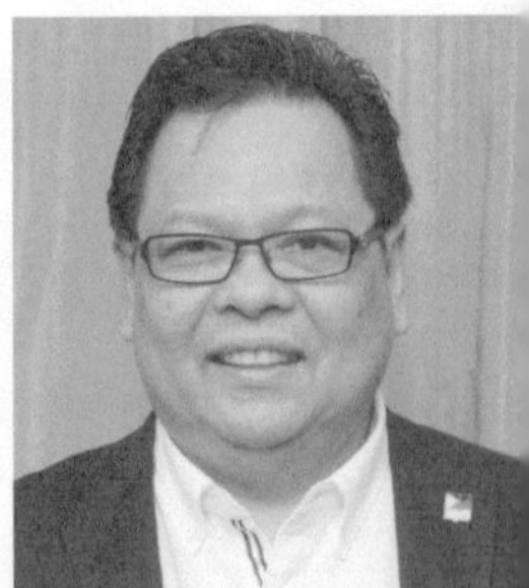
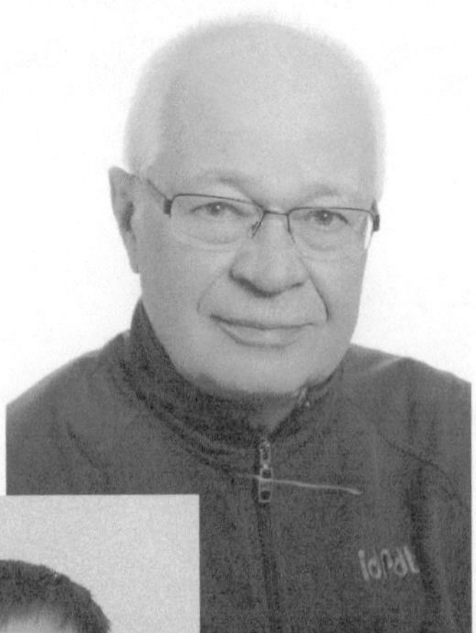
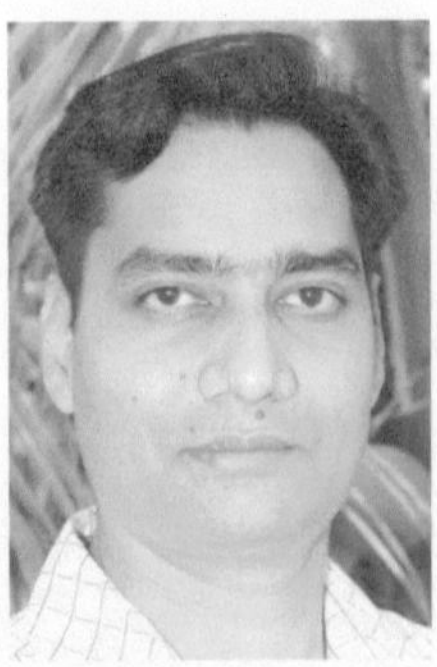
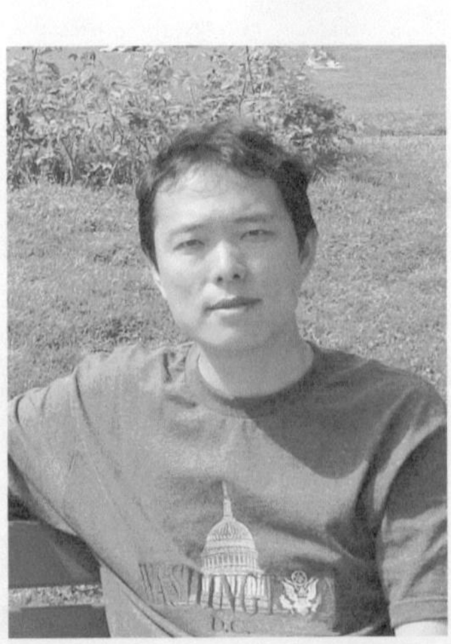
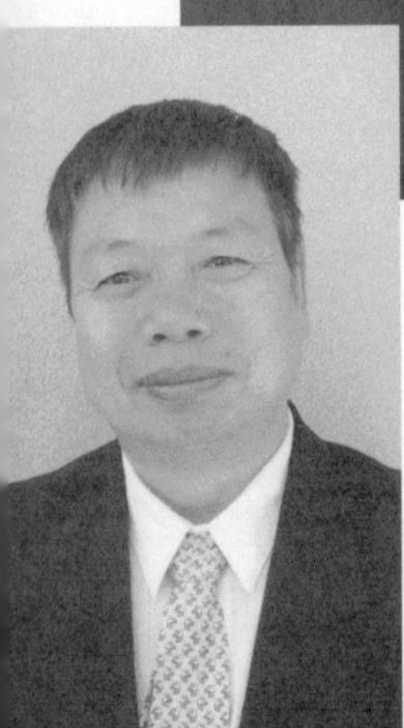
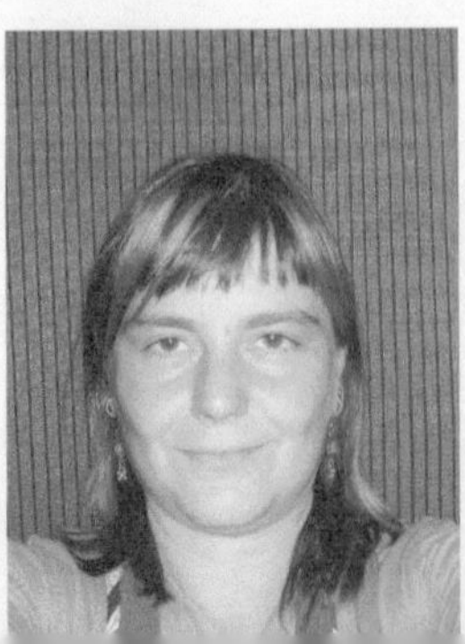

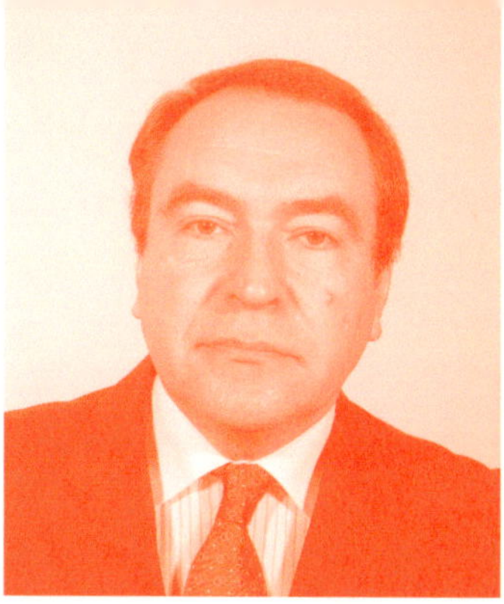
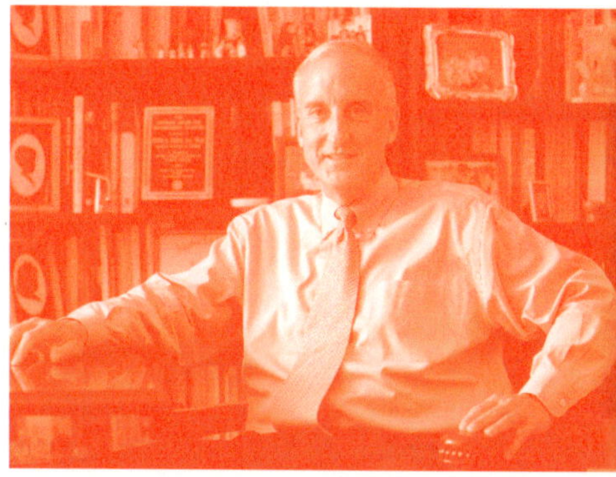
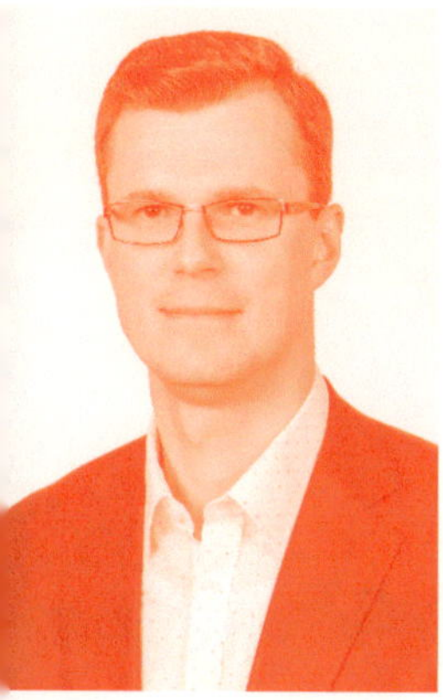
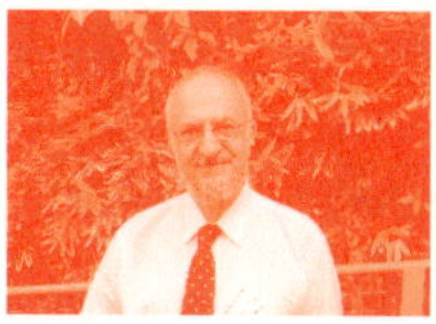
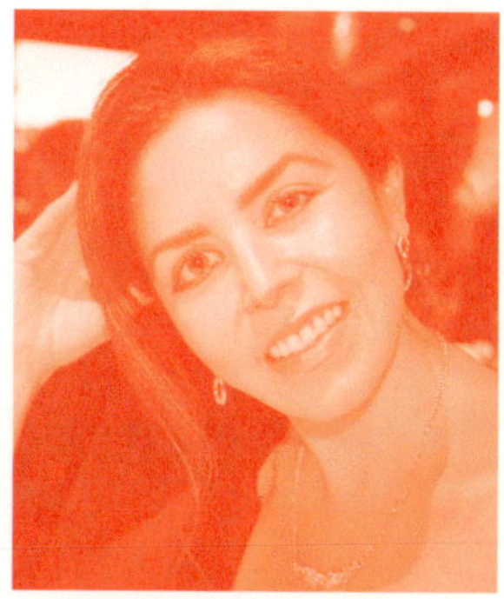

Supporting open minds since 2005

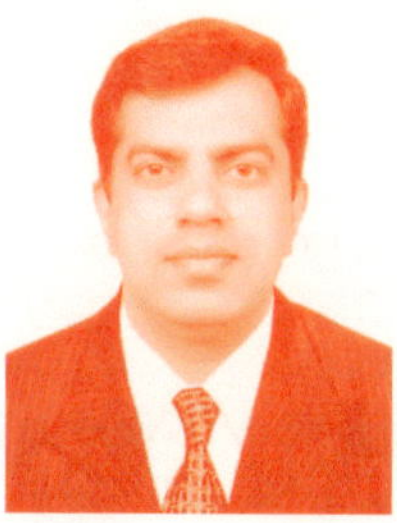
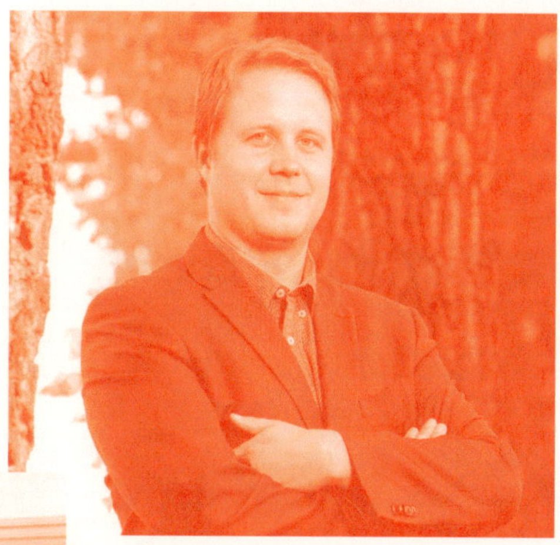
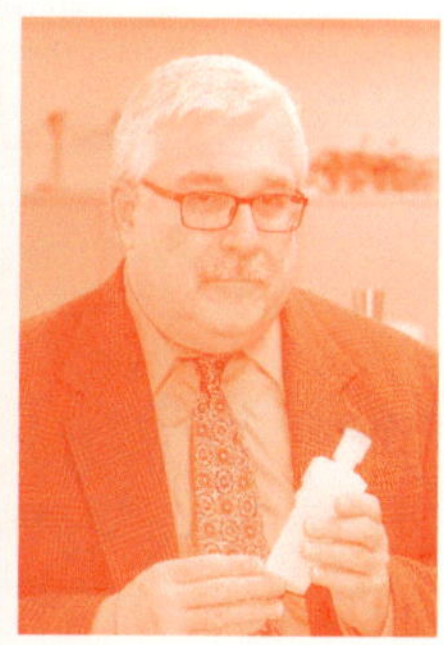
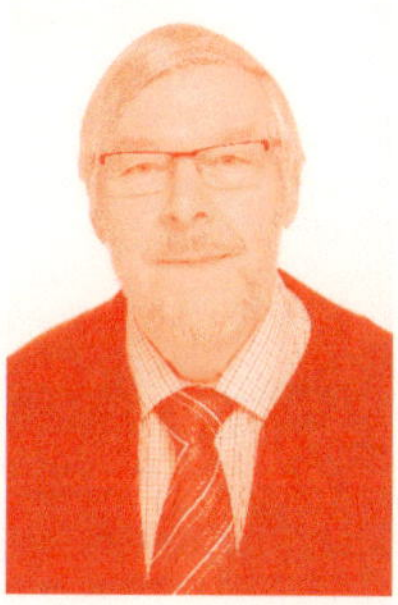
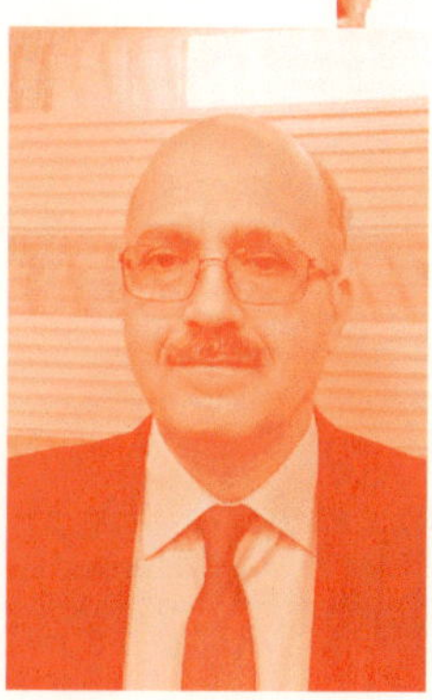
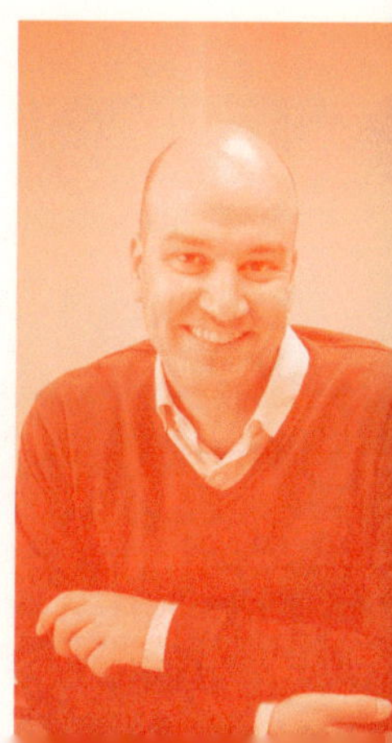
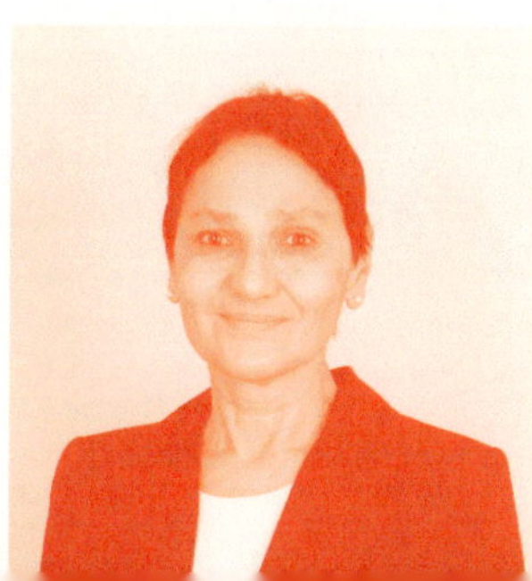

Assistive and Rehabilitation Engineering
http://dx.doi.org/10.5772/intechopen.77514
Edited by Yves Rybarczyk

Contributors
Sandra Sanchez-Gordon, Tania Calle-Jimenez, Janio Jadán-Guerrero, César Guevara, Patricia Acosta-Vargas, Jorge Luis Pérez Medina, Yves Rybarczyk, Subhasis Banerji, John Heng, Effie Chew, Christopher Wee Keong Kuah, Zhao Ling, Yan Ming Soh, Daphne Debby Menezes, Ponvignesh Ponnusamy, Gilbert Pradel, Nicolas Roche, Tong Li, Didier Pradon, Wilmer Esparza, Arian Ramón Aladro-Gonzalvo, Jonathan Baldeon, Sophia Ortiz, Pierre Boulanger, Peter Wood, Stephanie Schaeffer, Raj Padwal, Paolo Raggi, Willam Mott, Kaoru Sumi, Keigo Yabuki, Thomas James Tiam-Lee, Abdelkader Nasreddine Belkacem, Quentin Ferre, Shogo Hirai, Teruto Endo, Mengchun Xie, Keiko Tsujioka, Yves Philippe Rybarczyk

First published in London, United Kingdom, 2019 by IntechOpen
IntechOpen is the global imprint of INTECHOPEN LIMITED, registered in England and Wales, registration number: 11086078, 7th floor, 10 Lower Thames Street, London, EC3R 6AF, United Kingdom
Printed in Croatia

British Library Cataloguing-in-Publication Data
A catalogue record for this book is available from the British Library

Additional hard and PDF copies can be obtained from orders@intechopen.com

Assistive and Rehabilitation Engineering
Edited by Yves Rybarczyk
p. cm.
Print ISBN 978-1-78923-883-9
Online ISBN 978-1-78923-884-6
eBook (PDF) ISBN 978-1-78984-526-6

For EU product safety concerns:
IN TECH d.o.o. Prolaz Marije Krucifikse Kozulić 3, 51000 Rijeka, Croatia, info@intechopen.com or visit our website at intechopen.com.

Meet the editor

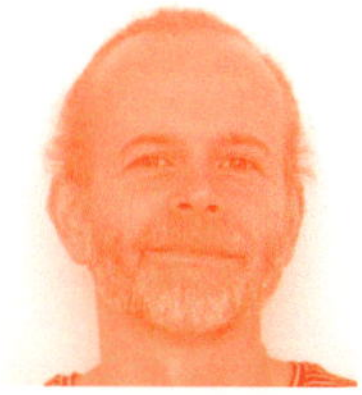

Yves Rybarczyk received a PhD degree in Robotics from the University of Evry, France, in 2004. His teaching and research activities focus on human–machine interaction and artificial intelligence. He was assistant professor at the Nova University of Lisbon between 2007 and 2015. Then, he moved to South America where he held the position of Associate Professor and Head of the Intelligent and Interactive Systems Laboratory at the Universidad de Las Américas until 2019. Currently, he is an associate professor at the University of Skövde, Sweden. He has participated in several projects on the modeling and development of complex and interactive systems. He is the author of over 80 scientific publications. Prof. Rybarczyk is a member of the steering committee of the International Summer Workshops on Multimodal Interfaces and a member of the editorial board of *IEEE Latin America Transactions*.

Contents

Preface

Rehabilitation enables people with motor, cognitive, and/or sensorial disabilities to regain functions and autonomy. However, over the past few years, there has been a reduction in healthcare providers to assist patients with impairments. Fortunately, this decline has been accompanied by an increase in information technologies to support health systems. This new paradigm brings promising perspectives, but also raises questions regarding the therapy assisted by computers. To address these issues, this book intends to clarify the multiple domains and application fields of medical engineering. The volume covers studies on rehabilitation and assistive technologies and the subtle difference between them. It especially focuses on the technical challenges and barriers regarding the nature of the disability: motor versus cognitive. It also provides a comprehensive approach to the recent advances in tele-health as a complementary medium to support the recovery process, and to enhance patients' empowerment and quality of life. Finally, it explains how artificial intelligence is impacting on tomorrow's medicine, especially in computer-aided diagnosis and self-rehabilitation.

The book is organized into four sections. The first section is an opening chapter introducing transdisciplinary considerations on interactive technologies. The second section is composed of three state-of-the-art studies. Chapter 2 is a systematic review of the design of a rehabilitation program adapted to technological support. Chapter 3 provides a state-of-the-art analysis of the development of usable and accessible telerehabilitation platforms. And Chapter 4 addresses the effect of feedback control loops on human information processing. The third section focuses on rehabilitation systems. Chapter 5 presents the case study of a rehabilitation application to support the recovery of patients after hip replacement surgery. Chapter 6 describes another therapeutic platform that makes use of virtual reality for remote cardiac rehabilitation. Chapter 7 proposes a new approach to restore independent living through the use of a wearable device and by taking advantage of the plasticity of the nervous system. The last section is dedicated to assistive systems. Chapter 8 describes an embedded device that assesses in real time the spatiotemporal gait pattern of patients after stroke injury. Chapter 9 proposes an innovative assistive system based on the cooperation between multi-agents and reinforcement learning. Finally, Chapter 10 completes the scope of the book by addressing cognitive issues on the design of cooperative games controlled by the brain–computer interface.

Yves Rybarczyk
Dalarna University,
Faculty of Data & Information Sciences,
Falun, Sweden

Section 1

Introduction

Chapter 1

Introductory Chapter: Transdisciplinary Considerations on Assistive and Rehabilitation Systems

Yves Rybarczyk

1. Introduction

Interacting with an assistive or rehabilitation device involves an adaptation of the cognitive and sensorimotor skills of the human being. This fact suggests that a successful development of such a system should imply transdisciplinary studies that consider both technological and psychological issues. **Figure 1** is a systematic representation that describes the phenomena that occur when an individual has to carry out an action mediated through an artefact [1]. Natural mechanisms enable the users to adapt their behaviours to the new situation. Nevertheless, this natural phenomenon presents certain limits and artificial implementations which could be necessary to reduce the gap between the human operator and the machine. The next two sections explain the processes that underlie the natural adaptation

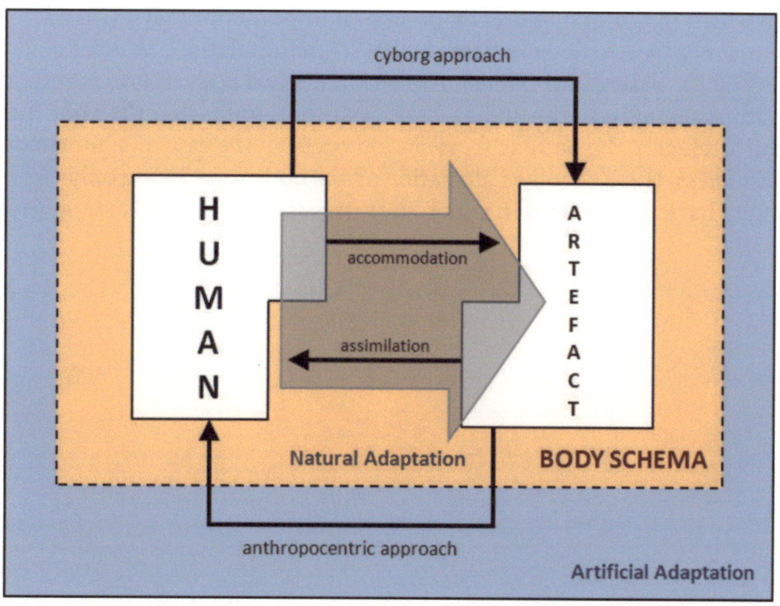

Figure 1.
Natural and artificial processes of adaptation that emerge or can be implemented in a context of human-machine interaction.

happening during the interaction with a tool and how this adaptation can be boosted by technological transformations of the artefact based on an anthropocentric approach.

2. Natural adaptation

According to Piaget [2] the adaptation to a new situation is supported by two complementary mechanisms described as assimilation and accommodation. This finding is based on studies in developmental psychology. Let us take the example of the action of banging, which is one of the favourite activities of the babies to explore the environment. The fact that the young children tend to replicate this same activity on different objects means that the scheme is assimilated by the individual. However, in certain situations it could be improper to reproduce a banging activity, in particular when the object is fragile like an egg. Since, it is not possible to apply the same scheme anymore, a transformation or accommodation of this pre-existing scheme is required. The same process seems to happen in adults when they have to complete an action mediated by an artefact [3]. According to the degree of familiarity with a new object and previous experience with properties of this object, the user will have to use former schemes (assimilation) and/or acquire new ones (accommodation) to properly interact with the artefact.

Once the appropriate schemes are established, a phenomenon of integration of the artefact into the body schema of the user can be observed. Neurophysiological evidences support this claim. Iriki et al. [4] recorded the activity of bimodal neurons of the monkey's brain that code for both visual and somatosensorial information of the animal's arm. The yellow, in **Figure 2** (left panel), is the space that triggers an activation of these neurons if a stimulus is placed in this area. If we let the monkey manipulate a rake for a relative short period of time, we can observe that the dimension of the area increases in such a way that it includes the length of the tool (**Figure 2**, right panel). A similar result was obtained in a more sophisticate setup, in which the animal indirectly perceived its body through a video screen [5]. These outcomes tend to demonstrate that, after manipulation, a device could be processed by the brain as an extension of the biological body. It is to mention that such neurons also exist in the human brain, which suggests that the same integration of an artefact in the body schema should occur in the case of a human operator.

Nevertheless, these proofs of alteration of the body schema are only demonstrated with basic equipment, in which the interaction is relatively straightforward.

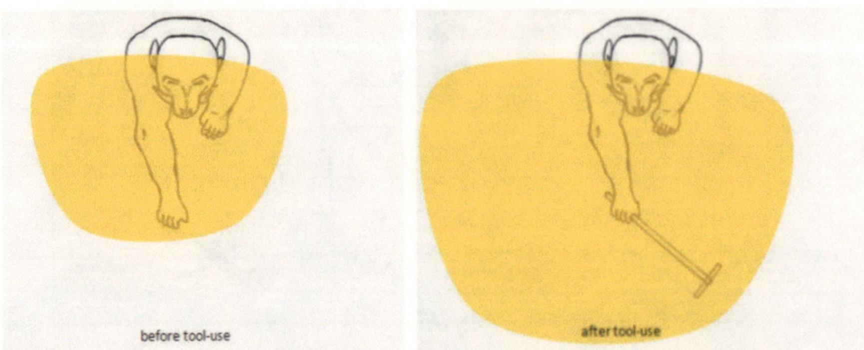

Figure 2.
Representation of the area (in yellow) coded by the bimodal neurons, before (left panel) and after (right panel) tool use.

It can be assumed that the natural adaptation would face its limits if the interactive system becomes more complex. In order to overcome these limitations, the next section presents successful case studies that implement an anthropocentric approach to promote an adaptation by assimilation.

3. Artificial adaptation

The application of an anthropocentric approach consists of modelling and implementing human-like behaviours in the assistive system. This method was applied in the context of the ARPH project, which consisted of developing a telerobot to increase the autonomy of motor disabled people [6]. The robot was composed of a robotic arm mounted on a mobile platform. The main limitation faced by the teleoperator was the reduced field of view of the robot's camera, which made difficult the remote control of the vehicle. Researches in experimental psychology show that walkers [7] or drivers [8] who have to change their direction tend to look to the inner part of the trajectory. It seems that the tangent point of the curve provides the individual with the most relevant information to guide the movement. This bio-inspired model of visuomotor anticipation over the locomotion was implemented on the assistive robot and compared to a machine-like behaviour [9]. The results show that the best performances in terms of velocity (completion time) and safety (number of collisions) are obtained with the human-like behaviour. Besides the raw performance, the quality of the robot control is also improved with the visuomotor anticipation, since the vehicle exhibits less jerky trajectories (**Figure 3**). This more natural way of driving suggests a better adaptation to the system when the machine replicates human features than when these characteristics are absent.

Another example of the benefit of the anthropocentric approach was observed with a fundamental law that characterises the human motricity, called 2/3 power law [10]. This law defines the relationship between the velocity and the curvature of the biological movements. It states that the angular velocity of the end effector is proportional to the two-thirds root of its curvature or, equivalently, that the instantaneous tangential velocity (v_t) is proportional to the third root of the radius of curvature (r_t), as described in Eq. (1). In other words, it means that the velocity of the movement decreases in the highly curved parts of the trajectory and increases when the trajectory becomes straighter. Rybarczyk and Carvalho [11] have

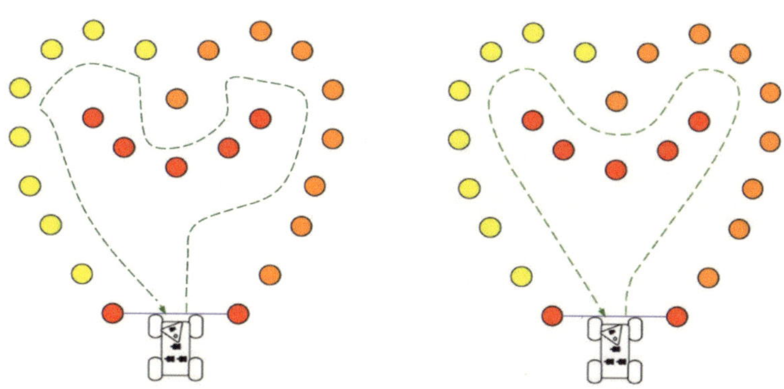

Figure 3.
Characteristics of the trajectories performed by a teleoperator when a machine-like (left panel) vs. a human-like (right panel) behaviour is implemented on a remote-controlled robot, to note the smoother path when the bio-inspired model is present.

demonstrated that a teleoperator adapts better to a remote-controlled robot when the 2/3 power law is implemented on the vehicle;

$$v_t = k r_t^{\frac{-1}{3}} \tag{1}$$

4. Conclusions

In line with this introductory chapter, the remaining of the book confirms that several scientific areas are involved in the development of assistive and rehabilitation systems. First of all, in terms of computer sciences, at least five specialties are represented: (i) software engineering, for the proper development of the applications; (ii) artificial intelligence, for the implementation and assessment of smart behaviours; (iii) health computing, to adapt the platform to the medical requirements; (iv) serious games, to increase the motivation of the patients; and (v) affective computing, to interpret the emotional state of the user. The second important area is human factors and ergonomics, which focus on (i) human-centred design, to make sure that the system is user-friendly, and (ii) user experience, to perform usability and accessibility studies. Finally, human sciences (psychology and neurosciences) and health sciences (paramedical fields) have a key role in (i) the design of experimental protocols, (ii) data analyses and (iii) adaptation of the traditional therapy to the new technologies. The next chapters address the interconnection between these complementary areas through the development of solutions for both assistive and rehabilitation purposes.

Author details

Yves Rybarczyk[1,2]

1 Dalarna University, Falun, Sweden

2 Universidad de Las Américas, Quito, Ecuador

*Address all correspondence to: y.rybarczyk@fct.unl.pt

References

[1] Rybarczyk Y, Hoppenot P, Colle E, Mestre D. Sensori-motor appropriation of an artefact: A neuroscientific approach. In: Inaki M, editor. Human Machine Interaction–Getting Closer. London: IntechOpen; 2012. pp. 187-212

[2] Piaget J. La Naissance de l'Intelligence chez l'Enfant. Paris, Lausanne: Delachaux et Niestlé; 1936

[3] Rabardel P. Les Hommes et les Technologies. Approche Cognitive des Instruments Contemporains. Paris: A. Colin; 1995

[4] Iriki A, Tanaka M, Iwamura Y. Coding of modified body schema during tool use by macaque postcentral neurons. Neuroreport. 1996;7:2325-2330

[5] Iriki A, Tanaka M, Obayashi S, Iwamura Y. Self-images in the video monitor coded by monkey intraparietal neurons. Neuroscience Research. 2001;**40**:163-173

[6] Colle E, Rybarczyk Y, Hoppenot P. ARPH: An assistant robot for disabled people. In: Proceedings of the IEEE International Conference on Systems, Man and Cybernetics 2002. Hammamet, Tunisia; 2002

[7] Grasso R, Glasauer S, Takei Y, Berthoz A. The predictive brain: Anticipatory control of head direction for the steering of locomotion. Neuroreport. 1996;7:1170-1174

[8] Land MF, Lee DN. Where we look when we steer? Nature. 1994;**369**:742-744

[9] Rybarczyk Y, Mestre D. Effect of temporal organization of the visuo-locomotor coupling on the predictive steering. Frontiers in Psychology. 2012;**3**:239. DOI: 10.3389/fpsyg.2012.00239

[10] Lacquaniti F, Terzuolo C, Viviani P. The law relating the kinematic and figural aspects of drawing movements. Acta Psychologica. 1983;**54**:115-130

[11] Rybarczyk Y, Carvalho D. Effect of the implementation of the two-third power law in teleoperation. In: Proceedings of the 7th International Conference on Applied Human Factors and Ergonomics. Orlando, FL, USA; 2016

Section 2

State of the Art

Chapter 2

Toward a Design of a Telerehabilitation Program for the Functional Recovery in Post-Hip Arthroplasty Patients

Wilmer Esparza, Arian Ramón Aladro-Gonzalvo, Jonathan Baldeon and Sophia Ortiz

Abstract

Telerehabilitation uses new information and communication technologies as an instrument to ensure a distant rehabilitation service. Patients who underwent hip replacement surgery are an excellent case study for the application of this technology. Post-surgical rehabilitation guidelines for hip arthroplasty are well known, and the correct application has a positive effect on the patients' prognosis. However, there are no complementary guidelines for physical therapy that could be used at a distance by patients through a computer platform. This chapter presents a systematic review about conventional physical therapy programs for hip arthroplasty. Based on this review, we proposed therapeutic exercises adapted to a low cost web-platform. In order to reach this objective we will present a brief review of the total hip arthroplasty, telemedicine, telerehabilitation and conventional physical therapy approaches.

Keywords: systematic review, telerehabilitation, web-platform, hip arthroplasty, physical therapy, functional recovery

1. Introduction

The technological advances and the greater access to knowledge networks have generated new treatment prototypes in the health field. An ongoing technological possibility that could complement the conventional physical therapy treatment is the telerehabilitation (TR) application. TR uses new information and communication technologies as an instrument to ensure a distant rehabilitation service. In addition, this tool optimizes recovery time and saves expenses in health services, benefitting both users and healthcare professionals.

The implementation of this technology is supported by: (i) health personnel; (ii) the impact on the patient's budget and the health system (lessening the number of medical appointments and therapy sessions, decreasing the time of hospitalization, and trips to the hospital); (iii) the expansion of medical care to distant or low-income populations; and (iv) the empowerment of the patient in the rehabilitation process.

Patients who underwent hip replacement surgery are an excellent case study for the application of this technology. Total hip arthroplasty (THA) involves replacing the skeletal surfaces of the hip joint (femoral head and acetabulum).

The coxofemoral joint is one of the most important joints in the human body, because it is fundamental for walking. The rehabilitation of these patients after surgery seeks to relieve pain, restore normal function and improve quality of life. Specifically, functional recovery plays an important role to engaging patient in activities of daily living (ADL).

Post-surgical rehabilitation guidelines for hip arthroplasty are well known, and the correct application has a positive effect on the patients' prognosis. However, there are no complementary guidelines for physical therapy that could be used at a distance by patients through a computer platform. A recent systematic review shows that the TR application in real time combined with a conventional physiotherapy program is more favorable than isolated treatment of musculoskeletal dysfunctions. Thus, the objective of this chapter was to report the main results of a systematic review about conventional physiotherapy programs for hip arthroplasty and to propose some exercises adapted to a low-cost TR platform for the functional recovery. We will present a brief review of the THA, telemedicine/TR, conventional physical therapy approaches, the methodology used to design the therapeutic intervention program adapted to the low-cost TR platform from a systematic literature review, and present the initial results about the implementation of some exercises.

2. Hip arthroplasty

The coxofemoral joint is formed by two articulated surfaces—the acetabulum and the femoral head—that are related to the hipbone and the femur, respectively. The THA consists of replacing the femoral head and the acetabulum with prosthesis. The surgery purpose is to reduce pain, improve mobility and quality of life the people with hip osteoarthrosis [1]. The type of THA to be performed will depend on the patient needs. In case of people with limited physical activity, a cemented THA is performed, while an uncemented THA is performed in people with high activity demands [2]. THA and knee arthroplasty are the most frequent surgical interventions in the USA, representing a high economic burden for the public and private health system [3, 4].

One of the main intervention shortcomings is related to the prosthesis lifetime, which depends on the amount of activity carried out with it. That means if the person performs activities with greater load on the lower limbs, the replacement period will be shorter compared to a person who performs less activity. Overall, the patients' progress after joint replacement is satisfactory. Nonetheless, a significant number of patients may present functional and balance limitations, even 1 year after surgery [5].

These limitations may imply deficits in the proprioceptive system that lead to altered pattern of movements (e.g., gait difficulties and poor postural control). Likewise, these alterations would disturb basic daily activities performance and patients' quality of life [6]. Therefore, balance and proprioception are key factors in the treatment to an integral rehabilitation [7]; since there is a positive association between equilibrium capacities and functional capacities [8].

3. Telemedicine and telerehabilitation

3.1 Telemedicine

The term telemedicine is used to describe the delivery of health care services, clinical information and patient education in all specialties. Telemedicine uses a wide variety of technologies (internet, mobile phones, electronic medical records...) to provide healthcare from distance [9]. It provides clinical information, allows consultations and helps communication between health professionals and patients, regardless the location of the patient. Therefore, telemedicine allows increasing access to specialized medical care. Remote patient monitoring happens regularly and certain interventions can be performed in real time rapidly and effectively [10]. Telemedicine can also be an instrument that helps patients and their caregivers get involved in their own care.

A large number of studies in a wide range of disciplines have bid to document the telemedicine effectiveness. It has been found that telemedicine is effective in the management of adult malnutrition [11]; asthma [12]; heart disease [13], diabetes—especially type 2 [14]; arterial hypertension [15] and multiple sclerosis [16]. In addition, positive clinical results have been presented for the patient follow-up and treatment in different situations such as: (1) burned [17]; (2) in palliative care [18]; (3) with acute cerebrovascular accident [19]; (4) with mental disorders [20]; (5) geriatric [21]; and (6) newborns, children and adolescents [22, 23].

Regardless the area in which telemedicine has been applied; different authors state general findings about its potential application. For instance, (1) It is a safe and feasible way to provide care and monitor certain groups of patients; (2) It leads to a decline in the number of visits to the hospital and decreases the length of stay in the hospital, therefore there is a reduction of costs in the health system; (3) Professionals and patients seem to follow and be satisfied when using the programs; and (4) It promotes self-management of the disease and adherence to treatment [24, 25]. Certainly, the increase usage of telemedicine could: (i) provide greater access to health services; (ii) offer the opportunity to carry out early interventions and even work on prevention; (iii) provide a constant follow-up, and (iv) involve the patient in the self-management of the disease.

3.2 Telerehabilitation

TR is a telemedicine form that provides remote support (temporary or permanent), evaluation and intervention to disabled people who need rehabilitation [26]. In the last decade TR has evolved due to the great reduction of costs in health services [27]. TR development has been pushed by several factors. Firstly, there is better access to specialized services and improved capacity for remote monitoring [28]. A second factor was the mobilization difficulties that people who require the service may face [26]. It has been shown that less than a third of patients discontinue outpatient rehabilitation 3 months after discharge [29]. In rural areas, transportation can be a burden due to less availability of public transportation or climatic factors. Thirdly, TR could defeat financial barriers for families with less purchasing power, since financing or using insurance in post-acute care is usually limited and expensive [26]. This reduces expenses for both, the user and the provider, because several patients can be treated by a single program at any time [27, 30]. Lastly, a key factor for TR progress is the connection between the healthcare provider and the patient, family members and the community which results in training improvement, which indirectly expands the health workforce [30].

The implementation of this technology is held by: (i) health personnel; (ii) the influence on the economy of the patients and the health system (decreased visits to the hospital and decreases the time of hospitalization); (iii) the ability of medical care to reach distant or low-income populations; and (iv) the autonomy of the patient in his rehabilitation process [26]. TR has been appropriate to: (i) complete pre-operative evaluations; (ii) analyze patterns of movement, gait; and (iii) prescribe orthopedic material [31]. These study trials showed favorable results, by not only improving physical health, reduction of fatigue, but also recovering mental health by the lessening of depressive symptoms. In addition, high levels of satisfaction and comfort were reported, as well as significant savings in time and travel costs of users [26, 31]. A recent study has aimed to develop a low-cost, online TR platform intended to evaluate and monitor patients after a total hip arthroplasty [32].

Despite all favorable aspects of the TR program implementation; there are still many challenges to face. The first challenge is to build a good relationship between the health provider and the patient. Many patients prefer to receive personalized and face-to-face care, lessening the possibilities of adopting this new form of approach. Elderly patients tend to have doubts about this kind of treatment method whereas it is extremely easy in young patients [30]. Developing an online application in smartphones could be one way to establish a relationship through TR [33]. These applications would allow a more direct, regular and personalized interaction with the patient.

There may also be safety problems, if the patient was alone during the session the patient could have an accident or when performing the movements wrongly increases the chances to get hurt [33, 34]. In order to avoid these situations, TR platforms should include links providing the necessary therapeutic information to prevent an accident or detect a wrong execution of the exercises. Likewise, the platform should be equipped with a control system able to allow the session to the patient, as well as disable it if necessary [32].

The incompatibility of systems and platforms between different operating system providers should also be taken care of. This issue has showed conflicts in the past when integrating the contents of clinical databases [34]. On the other hand, TR is limited when it comes to detecting fine movements or tremors, movements in certain planes [33], and emotional states of patients. However, recent studies show advances in the development of computer programming for facial gestures recognition that could be used in TR platforms [35].

4. Conventional physiotherapy

Physical therapy after a THA is essentially performed to improve patient's functionality through posture and gait training. Some of the main focuses during treatment are the hip range of motion (ROM), muscle strength, pain and edema. The control and improvement of these parameters allows the patient reintegration to the activities of daily life (ADL). This reintegration to the ADLs is accelerated when the rehabilitation process has an early start. Prompt physical therapy intervention helps reduce hospital stay, as well as costs to the health system [36].

Commonly the therapeutic intervention is classified as early, standard or late. The early intervention begins immediately after the surgery, and can be carried out on the same day or the next day. The standard phase begins either 1 or 2 days postoperative, while the late intervention begins after the second week post-surgery [36].

Depending on the patient activity, postoperative physical therapy can last between 8 to 24 weeks, divided into three or four phases. Stage I (peri-operative) lasts for 2 weeks where the focus is the education of the patient about their current condition (recommendations when doing certain movements, changes of position, training the walk with technical aids, etc.) and performing active mobility exercises in the appropriate ROM [37].

Stage II and III focus on muscle strengthening, load tissue adaptation and ROM recovery of the hip. This phase is usually distributed in two stages: the first lasts two to 8 weeks and the second between two and seven. Manual techniques can be used in this stage, but the progressive load with therapeutic exercise should be prioritized, in open and/or closed kinetic chain exercises, resistance exercises with elastic bands or different weights. In addition, stability and proprioception work should be included, with an emphasis on lumbopelvic and hip stability [37].

Stage IV concentrates on the ADL reintegration, it can last 2 weeks up to 2 months. The objective of this stage is to reinsert the patient to their normal setting (educational, work and/or sports activities). The approach is done through imitation of motor gestures accompanied by exercises of cardiovascular resistance and progressive strength. Cheatman and colleagues [37] estimate that after 4 months of intervention, the patient can return to his medium impact activities, such as the recreational walk. Six months after surgery, the patient can return to high impact activities or sports.

In general, physical therapy concentrates on muscle strength, patient education, gait retraining, and improvement of hip mobility. It is recommended to perform two sessions a day, since it has been demonstrated that in early stages function recovery occurs quicker [38]. Evidence also proves that rehabilitation programs, with at least three phases, have more beneficial effects for postoperative THA patients [37]. Finally, the fulfillment of the health team recommendations and complementary work at home are important in the rehabilitation process, accelerating the patient reintegration to their setting.

As we have shown, post-surgical rehabilitation guidelines for THA are well known, and their correct application has benefits on the patients′ prognosis. However, there are no complementary guidelines for physical therapy that could be used at a distance by patients through a computer platform. A recent systematic review shows that the TR application in real time combined with a conventional physiotherapy program is more favorable than isolated treatment of musculoskeletal dysfunctions [39].

5. Systematic review methodology

5.1 Data sources and searches

An electronic search was performed to identify relevant articles in: PubMed Meta-search (1950 to March, 2017), ScienceDirect (1990 to March, 2017), PEDro (1950 to March 2017), and Cochrane Database (2000 to March 2017). Key words relating to the domains was used: (1) type of exercise: "Join mobility exercise OR Functional exercise OR Therapeutic exercise OR Rehabilitation exercise OR Post-hospital Home Exercise"; (2) clinical term: "Total OR partial hip replacement, Total OR partial hip arthroplasty"; (3) type of document: "Position stand OR Clinical guide OR Systematic review OR Literature review OR Randomised controlled trials [RCTs];" (4) their combination.

5.2 Study selection

The reviewers followed a selection protocol, developed prior to the beginning of the review that included a checklist for inclusion and exclusion criterion (**Figure 1**). Articles were eligible for inclusion if they: (a) included passive or active specific exercises to strengthen the hip, enhance the static balance and/or restore whole joint movement; (b) were carried out on individuals of all age groups and sex with total or partial hip replacement; (c) consisted of self-administered home exercise programs or a program supervised by a physical therapist; (d) reported that a criterion for entry was total or partial hip replacement of 1 day after surgery and within 12 weeks to 8 months following surgery; (e) reported one of the following outcome

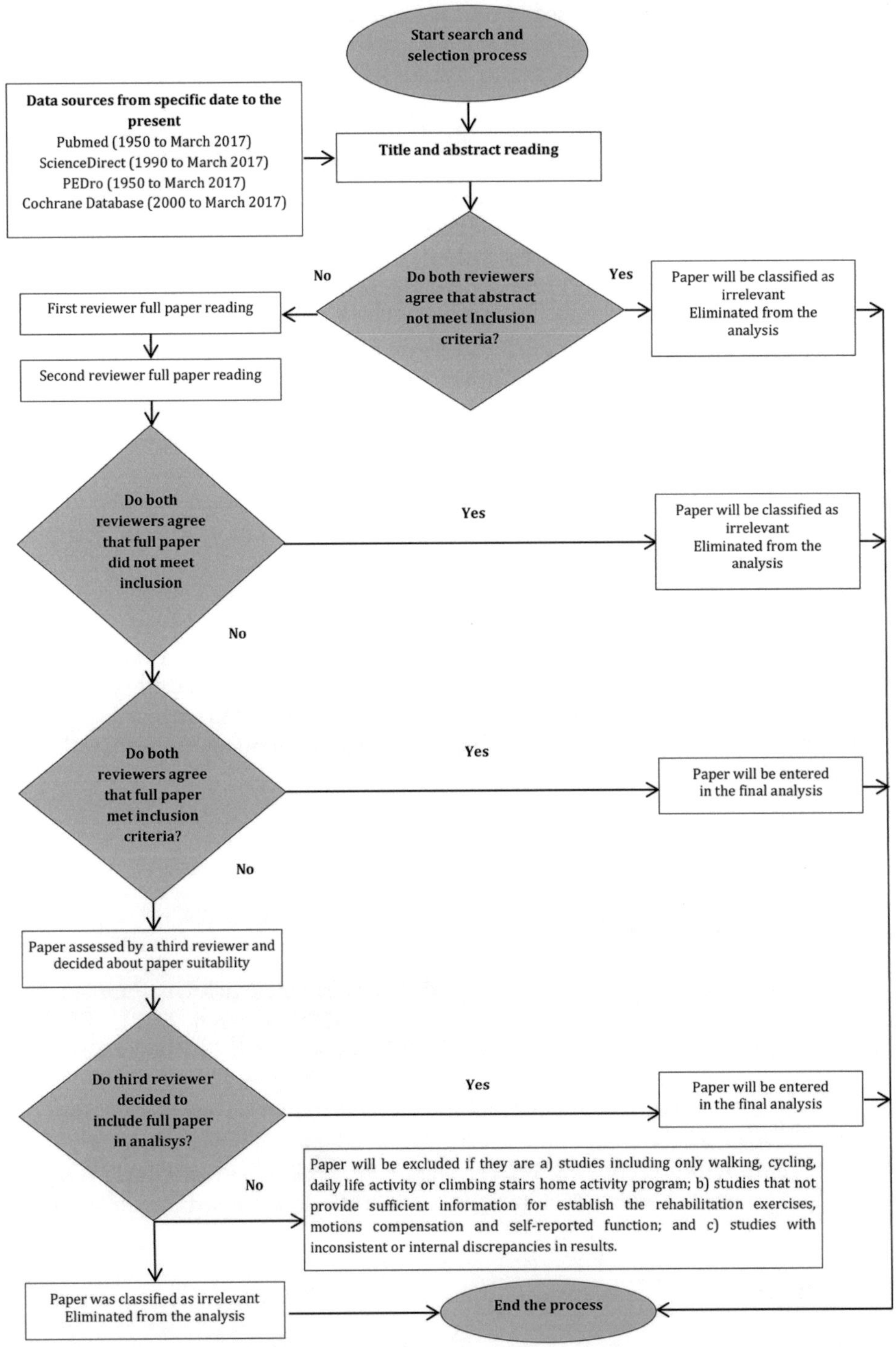

Figure 1.
Protocol used for studies selection.

measures: motions compensation and self-reported function; (f) were unpublished documents such as thesis, dissertations, and presentations in congresses; (g) peer-reviewed articles; and (h) were not restricted to any specific language.

Articles was excluded if they (a) included only walking, cycling, daily life activity or climbing stairs home activity program; (b) did not provide sufficient information for establish the rehabilitation exercises, motions compensation and self-reported function; and (c) showed inconsistent or internal discrepancies in results.

5.3 Data synthesis

The results were grouped under three characteristics: (1) specific passive or active exercises; (2) compensation of movements; and (3) self-report function. For specific exercises, the search focused on frequency (sets per hour); duration (time or repetitions per set); rest (recovery time); as well as the direction and speed of movement execution. Motion compensation analyzed the patient's position and the difficulties in performing the exercise. Finally, the function was related to the assessment of: (1) pain, (2) functional disability, (3) activities of daily life, and (4) perceived effort.

6. Results

6.1 Systematic review

The flow diagram using PRISMA statement depicts the different phases of systematic review [40]. It maps out the number of records identified, papers included/excluded, and the reasons for exclusions (**Figure 2**).

6.2 Program design

After inclusion and exclusion criteria application, only 19 studies were included for to design the program. These studies provided information about the elaboration of the program stages, as well as to establish the components and rehabilitation program objectives. The program stages are shown in **Figure 3**. For the instant, some exercises of the program have been validated in healthy people and patients with THA [32, 41].

6.2.1 Stage 1: acute rehabilitation

This stage starts immediately after the intervention. During this stage the main objectives are: (i) pain management; (ii) reduce postoperative edema; (iii) teach the patient the correct position and transfer changes; and (iv) activate and maintain lower limbs musculature (**Figure 4**).

Pain management: It has been agreed that the local application of cryotherapy yields to vasoconstriction and decay in the conduction speed of type C fibers. These properties help regulate pain, decrease postoperative edema and internal blood loss caused by osteosynthesis material attachment in the bone [46].

Activation and maintenance of the lower limb musculature: After a hip replacement surgery, isometric contraction decreases, leading to stability and functional complications. In order to maintain proper gait speed and prevent falls it is important to activate hip musculature (quadriceps, abductors and extensors). An effective muscular control helps restore patient function and independence [47].

Teaching positional changes and transfer of the patient: One of the goals to reach immediately after THA is the patient autonomy on the ADL, during the stay in the hospital and later at home. Training on positional and transfer changes is an education form, which decreases the stay length in the hospital and improves the patient recovery prognosis after the intervention [45].

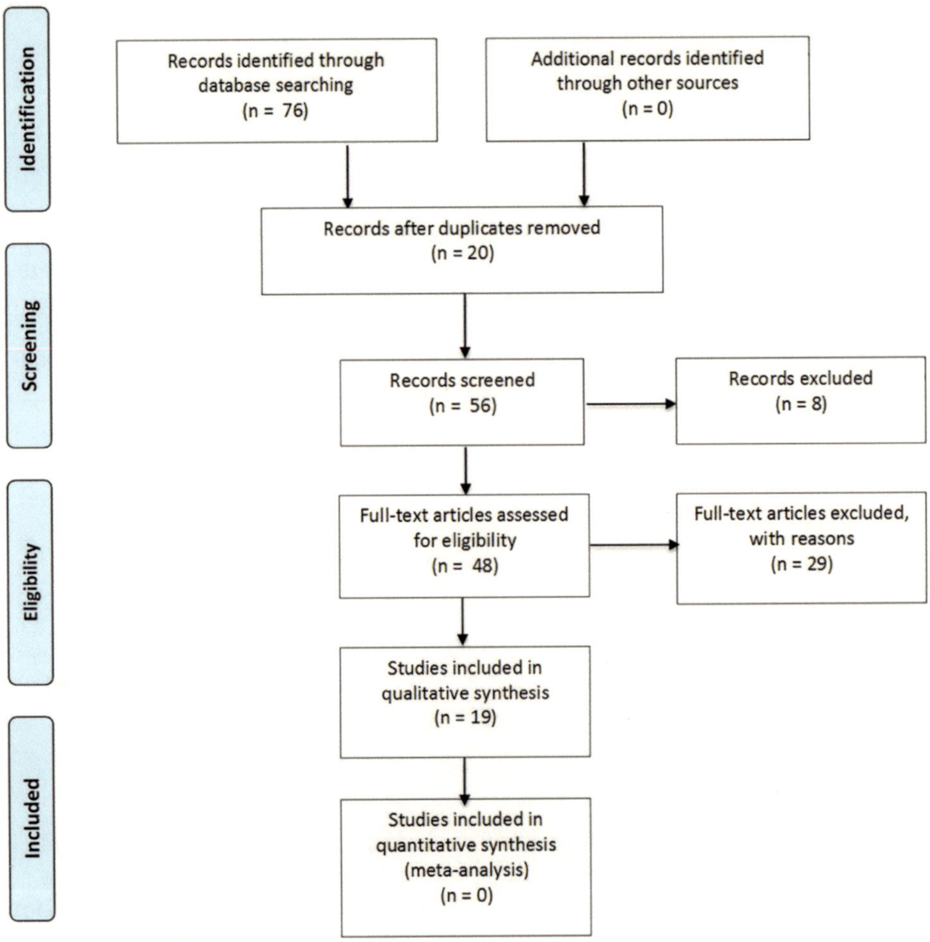

Figure 2.
Flow chart of systematic review process.

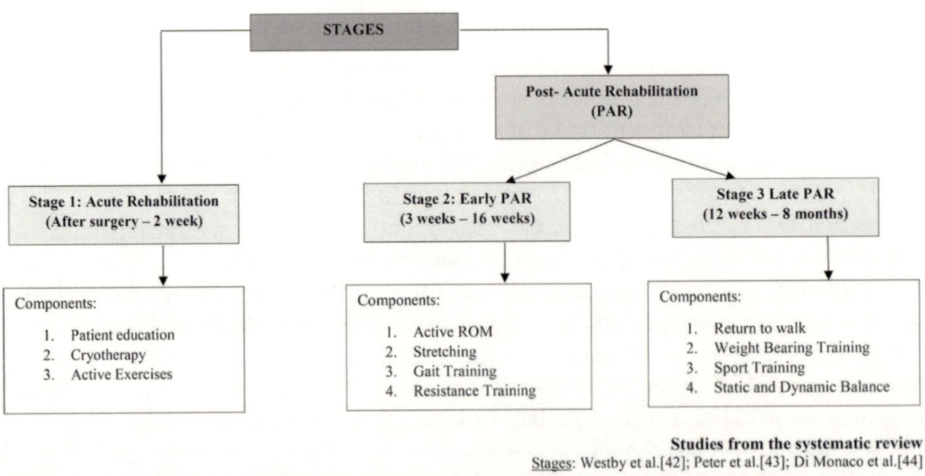

Figure 3.
Stages for acute and post-acute rehabilitation after total hip and knee arthroplasty [42–44].

6.2.2 Stage 2: early post-acute rehabilitation

This stage starts 3 weeks after surgery and lasts for 16 weeks. It focuses on recovering ROM and flexibility, as well as muscle and gait competence. This stage aims to prepare the lower limbs for the next stage of rehabilitation (**Figure 5**).

Active ROM mobility: After THA surgery the hip ROM decreases, caused by different factors such as post-surgical edema, protective muscular contraction, pain, capsular retractions, immobilization and patient's fear. This leads to gait deficits, static and dynamic postural instability, and limitation to perform ADL [49]. Consequently, patient function and independence are diminished.

Gait reeducation: Generally, gait patterns after THA surgery remain altered. For instance, there is Trendelemburg sign with a pelvis tilt towards the limb where the load is. This alteration is especially due to the gluteus medius dysfunction, which is severely affected during surgery [54]. The gait reeducation aims to recover the normal movement pattern. Visual, sensory and auditory feedback give information about the movement before it is automatized. It has been shown that reeducation with visual feedback promotes return to normal gait patterns in 3 weeks.

6.2.3 Stage 3: later post-acute rehabilitation

This stage lasts from week 12 to several months after surgery. The main objective on this stage is based on the functional reinsertion, gaining patient's autonomy in the DLAs (**Figure 6**).

Functional training: Since THA prevalence is higher in older adults the independence on DLA is conditioned to several factors. Among the most frequent factors there are physical deconditioning and geriatric syndromes (falls, gait disturbances, memory problems) [62]. Progressive strength training has been demonstrated to be essential for older populations, focused on reducing and preventing disability. Actually, muscle training leads to better static and dynamic postural control. The training strategies are based on leisure, recreational cooperative activities and based on the patient's ADL.

Postural control and dynamic stability: Postural control and dynamic stability depend on the proprioceptors integrity (articular, myotendinous, neuromuscular). Furthermore, after THA, the tissues integrity is lost, producing pain as well as

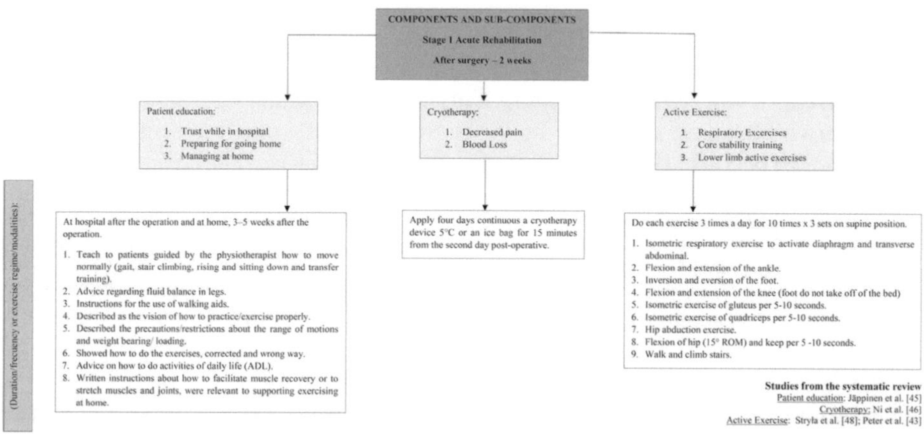

Figure 4.
Stage for acute rehabilitation after total hip and knee arthroplasty [43, 45, 46, 48].

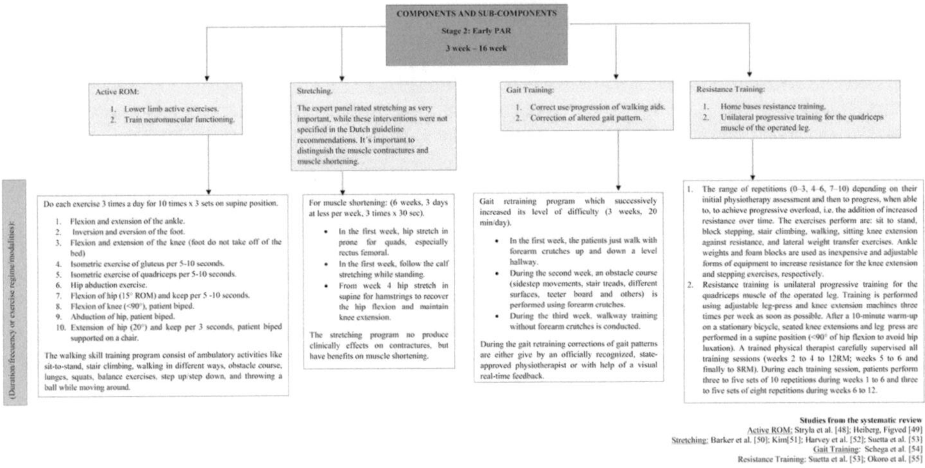

Figure 5.
Components and sub-components for the stage 2 [48–55].

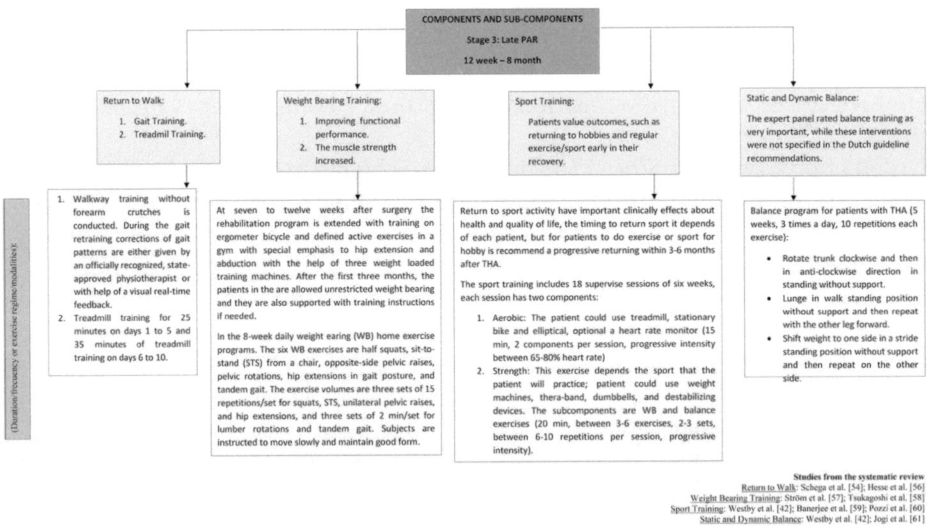

Figure 6.
Components and sub-components for the stage 3 [42, 54, 56–61].

muscle strength and ROM decrement's. This condition produces fear in the patient, leading to a high risk of falls, slowing down the gait, postural alterations and restrictions to perform the DLAs. Proprioceptive training through postural control improvement and dynamic stability aims to recover patient's function, normal gait pattern and quality of life [61].

7. Implementation design

This intervention program was designed as a low-cost online TR platform for self-motor rehabilitation and remote monitoring by health professionals, in order to enhance recovery in patients after hip replacement.

The Kinect camera was used as a natural user interface to capture some exercises performed by patients. The movement quality was evaluated in real time by an assessment module implemented according to a Hidden-Markov Model approach [63]. The exercise protocol was developed to supplement conventional physical therapy executed by patients at the hospital.

Before starting the exercise protocol, the platform requested the user to complete a questionnaire and an assessment about quality of life, functionality and DLAs. The questionnaire evaluates the patient's condition before undergoing the TR program. It is composed of three segments that inquire about pain, skin state and edema. Depending on user's responses, the platform allow the exercise program to be carried out during the session. The questionnaire served as a filter to access the program with the aim to avoid/control possible complications. Quality of life, functionality and DLAs were evaluated through the Oxford Scale for knee arthroplasty [64]. The questionnaire had to be completed at the beginning of each TR session while the functional evaluation at the end of each phase.

We will present the results of one [32], out of three preliminary studies, obtained after the implementation of some exercises proposed in this program. To record all movements a Kinect camera located approximately two meters away from the subjects was used.

Seven healthy subjects participated in the study comparing the assessment completed by four physiotherapists (PTs) with the evaluation performed by the TR platform algorithm.

The subjects were trained to perform a hip abduction movement, slow hip and knee flexion, hip extension and a sequence of steps forward, to the side and backwards. These sequences were repeated 11 times (one of them was used as a reference). The PTs had to follow an unknown script and it was randomized between participants (**Figure 7**).

The script was composed of six executions with normal ROM, two movements with an incorrect ROM and three compensatory movements. For each test, PTs were asked to evaluate all angles (ROM and compensations). The results of the

POSITION	MOVEMENT or EXERCISE	DESCRIPTION	TRAINING PATTERNS	OBSERVATIONS
Standing	Forward-sideway-backward sequence	Move the leg forward – return / – sideway- return/ and backward- return	- Sets: 3. -Repetitions per set: 10 - Rest between sets: 15 seconds	Return to initial position after each movement

Example

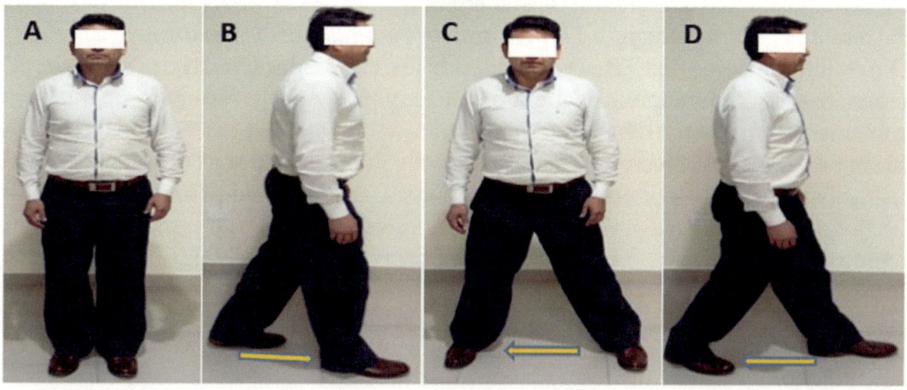

Figure 7.
Exercise for weight bearing training stage 3 (late PAR). (A) Initial position, (B) forward, (C) sideway, (D) backward.

evaluations were grouped into two categories that corresponded to incorrect or normal movement execution. The average of the four PTs scores were retained for the analyses. In case of a tie, the trial was discarded. Then, each average of this dichotomy variable (incorrect versus normal) were compared with the evaluation made by the algorithm. It was expected that the result would be different depending on the decision threshold.

The results showed that the algorithm corresponds in an 88% with the evaluation made by the PTs. There is certain variability in the performance of the assessment from one exercise to another. For example, the best results are obtained for the evaluation of the ROM for hip abduction and the forward and backward sequence (accuracy percentage > 90%).

The results of other studies were similar to these showing that it is possible to capture and analyze movement using a low cost system [32]. Consequently, the assessment of different types of movements, both in healthy people and in patients, has a high consistency rate among PTs and the system that is intended to be incorporated into a low-cost rehabilitation platform. A recent study validated the use of the Kinect within a TR system for THA (KiReS) [65]. This system allows PTs to define sets of exercises recorded in front of the Kinect. Successively, the patient executes the movement and his performance is compared to that of the PT. The movements analyzed were flexion, extension and abduction of the left and right hip. The unipodal equilibrium and squat movement executed with the lower left and right limb were also analyzed. The results showed a 91.88% consistency between the therapist's performance and that of the patient.

Our results are consistent with this study although our objective was to compare the simultaneous clinical assessment of several PTs with the system. However, the algorithms proposed in the three preceding studies not only evaluated and analyzed the limbs movement but also the compensatory movements. Patients often use compensatory strategies to facilitate movements [66]. Compensatory movements limit the limb affected functional recovery and can cause pain. This is the reason why a TR system should capture, limit and quantify the compensations. Compensatory movements adopted by patients create altered movement patterns that could limit the proper use of the affected limb in ADL [67, 68].

The Kinect camera works well especially when the user is facing the device, but the recognition of the skeleton from the top and side is not accurate. Moreover, in one of our studies the patient's clothing made it difficult to recognize the skeleton.

The TR could help solve accessibility limitations to rehabilitation services for many patients with THA. In addition, it can help reduce health care costs by allowing patients to empower themselves in their rehabilitation process. However, one of the biggest challenges is to convince the patient of the remote service. One study evaluated the feasibility of introducing a TR program for patients with THA, through a survey. The results indicated that TR in patients with THA is feasible from the perspective of access, feelings and preferences about technology [69]. Another study compared the implementation of a telerehabilitation program at home with a conventional rehabilitation program [70]. The results showed that the patients who got TR reached the same results for the evaluations on functional activities, exercises and patient education. Finally, a study comparing a TR program to a conventional THA program did not find significant differences in the results between the two programs [71].

8. Conclusions

The systematic review found 19 studies that explained the conventional physical therapy for THA. Commonly, the functional recovery is composed of three stages (acute, early and later rehabilitation). Based on this review, we designed exercises considering parameters such as ROM, coordination and compensation for a low cost TR web-platform. The exercises were evaluated at the same time by the PTs and by the platform. The algorithm used was able to recognize in real time the movements executed correctly and incorrectly in the three parameters mentioned above. The results showed compatibility between 88 and 91% (according to the movement assessed) between the TR system and the clinical assessment performed by the PTs. Furthermore, it is important to note that not all exercises applied in conventional physical therapy are possible to replicate in a TR system. This is due to the limitations of the movement capture by low-cost systems. Thus, for the moment this system can be used as a complement to conventional physical therapy. We can conclude that some exercises used as well as the movement analysis system can be implemented in a low-cost TR platform.

Acknowledgements

This research has been partially supported by the Consorcio Ecuatoriano para el Desarrollo de Internet Avanzado (CEDIA), Grant CEPRA-XI-2017-2115.

Conflict of interest

No conflicts of interest have been reported by the authors or by any individuals in control of the content of this article.

Author details

Wilmer Esparza[1,2,3*], Arian Ramón Aladro-Gonzalvo[1], Jonathan Baldeon[2] and Sophia Ortiz[2]

1 Facultad de Enfermería, Pontificia Universidad Católica del Ecuador, Quito, Ecuador

2 School of Physical Therapy, Universidad de Las Américas, Quito, Ecuador

3 Intelligent and Interactive Systems Lab, Universidad de Las Américas, Quito, Ecuador

*Address all correspondence to: wilmer.esparza@udla.edu.ec

References

[1] Almeida GJ, Khoja SS, Piva SR. Physical activity after total joint arthroplasty: A narrative review. Open Access Journal of Sports Medicine. 2018;**9**:55-68. DOI: 10.1002/acr.2271

[2] Brotzman SB, Manske RC. Clinical Orthopaedic Rehabilitation: A Team Approach. 4th ed. Philadelphia, PA: Elsevier; 2018. p. 560

[3] Abdulkarim A, Ellanti P, Motterlini N, Fahey T, O'Byrne JM. Cemented versus uncemented fixation in total hip replacement: A systematic review and meta-analysis of randomized controlled trials. Orthopedic Reviews. 2013;**5**(1):34-44. DOI: 10.4081/or.2013.e8

[4] Fusco F, Campbell H, Barker K. Rehabilitation after resurfacing hip arthroplasty: Cost-utility analysis alongside a randomized controlled trial. Clinical Rehabilitation. 2019:1-12. DOI: 10.1177/0269215519827628

[5] Majewski M, Bischoff-Ferrari HA, Grüneberg C, Dick W, Allum JHJ. Improvements in balance after total hip replacement. The Journal of Bone and Joint Surgery. 2005;**87**(10):1337-1343. DOI: 10.1302/0301-620X.87B10.16605

[6] Sharma M, Behera P, Sen RK, Aggarwal S, Tripathy SK, Prakash M, et al. Total hip arthroplasty for arthritis following acetabular fractures-evaluation of radiological, functional and quality of life parameters. Journal of Clinical Orthopaedics and Trauma. 2019;**10**(1):131-137. DOI: 10.1016/j.jcot.2017.10.017

[7] Judd DL, Winters JD, Stevens-Lapsley JE, Christiansen CL. Effects of neuromuscular reeducation on hip mechanics and functional performance in patients after total hip arthroplasty: A case series. Clinical Biomechanics. 2016;**32**:49-55. DOI: 10.1016/j.clinbiomech.2015.12.008

[8] Shimada H, Obuchi S, Kamide N, Shiba Y, Okamoto M, Kakurai S. Relationship with dynamic balance function during standing and walking. American Journal of Physical Medicine & Rehabilitation. 2003;**82**(7):511-516. DOI: 10.1097/01.PHM.0000064726.59036.CB

[9] Maheu MM, Whitten P, Allen A, editors. E-health, Telehealth, and Telemedicine: A Guide to Start-up and Success. 1st ed. New York, NY: Jossey-Bass; 2007. p. 400

[10] Lesher AP, Shah SR. Telemedicine in the perioperative experience. Seminars in Pediatric Surgery. 2018;**27**(2):102-106. DOI: 10.1053/j.sempedsurg.2018.02.007

[11] Marx W, Kelly JT, Crichton M, Craven D, Collins J, Mackay H, et al. Is telehealth effective in managing malnutrition in community-dwelling older adults? A systematic review and meta-analysis. Maturitas. 2018;**111**:31-46. DOI: 10.1016/j.maturitas.2018.02.012

[12] Kew KM, Cates CJ. Remote versus face-to-face check-ups for asthma. Cochrane Database of Systematic Reviews. 2016;**4**:1-59. DOI: 10.1002/14651858.CD011715.pub2

[13] Raikhelkar J, Raikhelkar JK. The impact of telemedicine in cardiac critical care. Critical Care Clinics. 2015;**31**(2):305-317. DOI: 10.1016/j.ccc.2014.12.008

[14] Su D, Zhou J, Kelley MS, Michaud TL, Siahpush M, Kim J, et al. Does telemedicine improve treatment outcomes for diabetes? A meta-analysis of results from 55 randomized controlled trials. Diabetes Research and Clinical Practice. 2016;**116**:136-148. DOI: 10.1016/j.diabres.2016.04.019

[15] Zhou R, Cao Y, Zhao R, Zhou Q, Shen J, Zhou Q, et al. A novel cloud based auxiliary medical system for hypertension management. Applied Computing and Informatics 2018; (in press), Corrected Proof. DOI: 10.1016/j.aci.2017.10.002

[16] D'hooghe M, Van Gassen G, Kos D, Bouquiaux O, Cambron M, Decoo D, et al. Improving fatigue in multiple sclerosis by smartphone-supported energy management: The MS TeleCoach feasibility study. Multiple Sclerosis and Related Disorders. 2018;**22**:90-96. DOI: 10.1016/j.msard.2018.03.020

[17] Hickey S, Gomez J, Meller B, Schneider JC, Cheney M, Nejad S, et al. Interactive home telehealth and burns: A pilot study. Burns. 2017;**43**(6):1318-1321. DOI: 10.1016/j.burns.2016.11.013

[18] Bonsignore L, Bloom N, Steinhauser K, Nichols R, Allen T, Twaddle M, et al. Evaluating the feasibility and acceptability of a telehealth program in a rural palliative care population: Tapcloud for palliative care. Journal of Pain and Symptom Management. 2018;**56**(1):7-14. DOI: 10.1016/j.jpainsymman.2018.03.013

[19] Arba F, Piccardi B, Baldereschi M, Ricci S, Inzitari D. Telemedicine for acute ischaemic stroke. Cochrane Database of Systematic Reviews. 2016;**2**:1-7. DOI: 10.1002/14651858.CD012070

[20] Stratton E, Lampit A, Choi I, Calvo RA, Harvey SB, Glozier N. Effectiveness of eHealth interventions for reducing mental health conditions in employees: A systematic review and meta-analysis. PLoS ONE. 2017;**12**(12):e0189904. DOI: 10.1371/journal.pone.0189904

[21] Salles N, Lafargue A, Cressot V, Glenisson L, Barateau M, Thiel E, et al. Global geriatric evaluation is feasible during interactive telemedicine in nursing homes. European Research in Telemedicine/La Recherche Européenne en Télémédecine. 2017;**6**(2):59-65. DOI: 10.1016/j.eurtel.2017.06.002

[22] Tan K, Lai NM. Telemedicine for the support of parents of high risk newborn infants. Cochrane Database of Systematic Reviews. 2012;**6**:1-17. DOI: 10.1002/14651858.CD006818.pub2

[23] Myers KM, Palmer NB, Geyer JR. Research in child and adolescent telemental health. Child and Adolescent Psychiatric Clinics. 2011;**20**(1):155-171. DOI: 10.1016/j.chc.2010.08.007

[24] Flodgren G, Racha A, Farmer AJ, Inzitari M, Shepperd S. Interactive telemedicine: Effects on professional practice and health care outcomes. Cochrane Database of Systematic Reviews. 2015;**9**:1-555. DOI: 10.1002/14651858.CD002098.pub2

[25] Huang TT, Sung CC, Wang WS, Wang BH. The effects of the empowerment education program in older adults with total hip replacement surgery. Journal of Advanced Nursing. 2017;**73**(8):1848-1861. DOI: 10.1111/jan.13267

[26] Gregory P, Alexander J, Satinsky J. Clinical telerehabilitation: Applications for physiatrists. PM & R: The Journal of Injury, Function, and Rehabilitation. 2011;**3**:647-656. DOI: 10.1016/j.pmrj.2011.02.024

[27] Rogante M, Grigioni M, Cordella D, Giacomozzi C. Ten years of telerehabilitation: A literature overview of technologies and clinical applications. Neuropsychological Rehabilitation. 2010;**27**(4):287-304. DOI: 10.3233/NRE-2010-0612

[28] Ackerman MJ, Filart R, Burgess LP, Lee I, Poropatich RK. Developing next-generation telehealth tools and technologies: Patients, systems and data perspectives. Telemedicine Journal and E-Health. 2010;**16**(1):93-95. DOI: 10.1089/tmj.2009.0153

[29] McHugh GA, Campbell M, Luker KA. Predictors of outcomes of recovery following total hip replacement surgery: A prospective study. Bone & Joint research. 2013;**2**(11):248-254. DOI: 10.1302/2046-3758.211.2000206

[30] Morales-Vidal S, Ruland S. Telemedicine in stroke care and rehabilitation. Topics in Stroke Rehabilitation. 2013;**20**(2):101-107. DOI: 10.1310/tsr2002-101

[31] Russell TG, Blumke R, Richardson B, Truter P. Telerehabilitation mediated physiotherapy assessment of ankle disorders. Physiotherapy Research International. 2010;**15**(3):167-175. DOI: 10.1002/pri.471

[32] Rybarczyk Y, Pérez Medina JL, Leconte L, Jimenes K, González M, Esparza D. Implementation and assessment of an intelligent motor tele-rehabilitation platform. Electronics. 2019;**8**(58):1-24. DOI: 10.3390/electronics8010058

[33] Lemaire ED, Boudrias Y, Greene G. Low-bandwidth, internet-based video conferencing for physical rehabilitation consultations. Journal of Telemedicine and Telecare. 2001;**7**:82-89. DOI: 10.1258/1357633011936200

[34] Schein RM, Schmeler MR, Brienza D, Saptono A, Parmanto B. Development of a service delivery protocol used for remote wheelchair consultation via telerehabilitation. Telemedicine and e-Health. 2008;**14**(9):932-938. DOI: 10.1089/tmj.2008.0010

[35] Vanderdonckt J Roselli P, Pérez-Medina JL. FTL, an articulation-invariant stroke gesture recognizer with controllable position, scale, and rotation invariances. In: Proceedings of the 20th ACM International Conference on Multimodal Interaction. 2018. pp. 125-134. DOI: 10.1145/3242969.3243032

[36] Masaracchio M, Hanney WJ, Liu X, Kolber M, Kirker K. Timing of rehabilitation on length of stay and cost in patients with hip or knee joint arthroplasty: A systematic review with meta-analysis. PLoS One. 2017;**12**(6):e0178295. DOI: 10.1371/journal.pone.0178295

[37] Cheatham S, Mokha M, Lee M. Postoperative rehabilitation after hip resurfacing: A systematic review. Journal of Sport Rehabilitation. 2016;**25**(2):181-189. DOI: 10-1123/jsr.2014-0270

[38] Di Monaco MD, Castiglioni C. Which type of exercise therapy is effective after hip arthroplasty? A systematic review of randomized controlled trials. European Journal of Physical and Rehabilitation Medicine. 2013;**49**(6):893-907. Available from: https://www.semanticscholar.org/paper/Which-type-of-exercise-therapy-is-effective-after-A-Monaco-Castiglioni/ee933004cc9bab9464d81a1a566cf70ed7708814

[39] Cottrell MA, Galea OA, O'Leary SP, Hill AJ, Russell TG. Real-time telerehabilitation for the treatment of musculoskeletal conditions is effective and comparable to standard practice: A systematic review and meta-analysis. Clinical Rehabilitation. 2017;**31**(5):625-638. DOI: 10.1177/0269215516645148

[40] Moher D, Liberati A, Tetzlaff J, Altman DG. The PRISMA group. Preferred reporting items for systematic reviews and meta-analyses: The PRISMA statement. International Journal of Surgery. 2010;**8**(5):336-341. DOI: 10.1371/journal.pmed.1000097

[41] Rybarczyk Y, Deters JK, Cointe C, Esparza D. Smart web-based platform to support physical rehabilitation. Sensors (Basel, Switzerland). 2018;**18**(5):1344. DOI: 10.3390/s18051344

[42] Westby MD, Brittain A, Backman CL. Expert consensus on best practices for post–acute rehabilitation after

total hip and knee arthroplasty: A Canada and United States Delphi study. Arthritis Care and Research. 2014;**66**(3):411-423. DOI: 10.1002/acr.22164

[43] Peter W, Nelissen R, Vlieland T. Guideline recommendations for post-acute postoperative physiotherapy in total hip and knee arthroplasty: Are they used in daily clinical practice? Musculoskeletal Care. 2014;**12**(3): 125-131. DOI: 10.1002/msc.1067

[44] Di Monaco M, Vallero F, Tappero R, Cavanna A. Rehabilitation after total hip arthroplasty: A systematic review of controlled trials on physical exercise programs. European Journal of Physical and Rehabilitation Medicine. 2009;**45**(3):303-317. Available from: https://pdfs.semanticscholar.org/3d3f/3d6ccf4e43b9e1a53537ef9ce9ea6c75fa5f.pdf

[45] Jäppinen AM, Hämäläinen H, Kettunen T, Piirainen A. Postoperative patient education in physiotherapy after hip arthroplasty: Patient perspective. Musculoskeletal Care. 2017;**15**(2): 150-157. DOI: 10.1002/msc.1153

[46] Ni S, Jiang WT, Guo L, Jin YH, Jiang TL, Zhao Y, et al. Cryotherapy on postoperative rehabilitation of joint arthroplasty. Knee Surgery, Sports Traumatology, Arthroscopy. 2015;**23**(11):3354-3361. DOI: 10.1007/s00167-014-3135-x

[47] Frost K, Bertocci G, Wassinger C, Munin M, Burdett R, Fitzgerald S. Isometric performance following total hip arthroplasty and rehabilitation. Journal of Rehabilitation Research and Development. 2006;**43**(3):435-444. DOI: 10.1682/JRRD.2005.06.0100

[48] Stryła W, Pogorzała A, Rogala P, Nowakowski A. Algorithm of physical therapy exercises following total hip arthroplasty. Polish Orthopaedics and Traumatology. 2013;**78**:33-39. Available from: https://europepmc.org/abstract/med/23306317

[49] Heiberg K, Figved W. Physical functioning and prediction of physical activity after Total hip arthroplasty: Five-year follow up of a randomized controlled trial. Arthritis Care & Research (Hoboken). 2016;**68**(4): 454-462. DOI: 10.1002/acr.22679

[50] Barker K, Newman M, Hughes T, Sackley C, Pandit H, Kiran A, et al. Recovery of function following hip resurfacing arthroplasty: A randomized controlled trial comparing an accelerated versus standard physiotherapy rehabilitation programme. Clinical Rehabilitation. 2013;**27**(9):771-784. DOI: 10.1177/0269215513478437

[51] Kim J. The frequency of hamstring stretches required to maintain knee extension range of motion following an initial six-week stretching programme. [thesis] Auckland: University of Technology; 2012. Available from: http://aut.researchgateway.ac.nz/bitstream/handle/10292/5292/kimj.pdf?sequence=3.

[52] Harvey L, Katalinic O, Herbert R, Moseley A, Lannin N, Schurr K. Stretch for the treatment and prevention of contractures. Cochrane Database of Systematic Reviews. 2017;(1):1-181. DOI: 10.1002/14651858.CD007455.pub3

[53] Suetta C, Magnusson S, Rosted A, Aagaard P, Jakobsen A, Larsen L, et al. Resistance training in the early postoperative phase reduces hospitalization and leads to muscle hypertrophy in elderly hip surgery patients-a controlled, randomized study. Journal of the American Geriatrics Society. 2004;**52**(12):2016-2022. DOI: 10.1111/j.1532-5415.2004.52557.x

[54] Schega L, Bertram D, Fölsch C, Hamacher D, Hamacher D. The influence of visual feedback on the

mental representation of gait in patients with THR: A new approach for an experimental rehabilitation strategy. Applied Psychophysiology and Biofeedback. 2014;**39**(1):37-43. DOI: 10.1007/s10484-014-9239-8

[55] Okoro T, Whitaker R, Gardner A, Maddison P, Andrew J, Lemmey A. Does an early home-based progressive resistance training program improve function following total hip replacement? Results of a randomized controlled study. BMC Musculoskeletal Disorders. 2016;**17**:173. DOI: 10.1186/s12891-016-1023-x

[56] Hesse S, Werner C, Seibel H, von Frankenberg S, Kappel EM, Kirker S, et al. Treadmill training with partial body-weight support after total hip arthroplasty: A randomized controlled trial. Archives of Physical Medicine and Rehabilitation. 2008;**84**:1767-1773. DOI: 10.1016/S0003-9993(03)00434-9

[57] Ström H, Huss K, Larsson S. Unrestricted weight bearing and intensive physiotherapy after uncemented total hip arthroplasty. Scandinavian Journal of Surgery. 2006;**95**(1):55-60. DOI: 10.1177/145749690609500111

[58] Tsukagoshi R, Tateuchi H, Fukumoto Y, Ibuki S, Akiyama H, So K, et al. Functional performance of female patients more than 6 months after total hip arthroplasty shows greater improvement with weight-bearing exercise than with non-weight-bearing exercise. Randomized controlled trial. European Journal of Physical and Rehabilitation Medicine. 2014;**50**(6): 665-675. Available from: https://europepmc.org/abstract/med/25051209

[59] Banerjee M, Bouillon B, Banerjee C, Bäthis H, Lefering R, Nardinj M, et al. Sports activity after total hip resurfacing. The American Journal of Sports Medicine. 2010;**38**(6):1229-1236. DOI: 10.1177/0363546509357609

[60] Pozzi F, Madara K, Zeni K. A six-week supervised exercise and educational intervention after total hip arthroplasty: A case series. International Journal of Sports Physical Therapy. 2017;**12**(2):259-272. Available from: https://www.ncbi.nlm.nih.gov/pmc/articles/PMC5380869/

[61] Jogi P, Zecevic A, Overend T, Spaulding S, Kramer J. Force-plate analyses of balance following a balance exercise program during acute post-operative phase in individuals with total hip and knee arthroplasty: A randomized clinical trial. SAGE Open Medicine. 2016;**4**:1-9. DOI: 10.1177/2050312116675097

[62] Inouye SK, Studenski S, Tinetti M, Kuchel GA. Geriatric syndromes: Clinical, research and policy implications of a core geriatric concept. Journal of the American Geriatrics Society. 2007;**55**(5):780-791. DOI: 10.1111/j.1532-5415.2007.01156.x

[63] Rybarczyk Y, Cointe C, Gonçalves T, Minhoto V, DetersJ K, Villarreal S, et al. On the use of natural user interfaces in physical rehabilitation: A web-based application for patients with hip prosthesis. Journal of Science and Technology of the Arts. 2018;**10**(2):2-15. DOI: 10.7559/citarj.v10i1.402

[64] Dawson J, Fitzpatrick R, Frost S, Gundie R, McLardy-Smith P, Murray D. Evidence for the validity of a patient based instrument for assesment of outcome after revision hip replacement. The Journal of bone and joint surgery. British. 2001;**83**(8):1125-1129. DOI: 10.1302/0301-620X.83B8.11643

[65] Anton D, Nelson M, Russell T, Goñi A, Illarramendi A. Validation of a Kinect-based telerehabilitation system with total hip replacement patients. Journal of Telemedicine and Telecare. 2016;**22**(3):192-197. DOI: 10.1177/1357633X15590019

[66] Jones TA. Motor compensation and its effects on neural reorganization after stroke. Nature Reviews Neuroscience. 2017;**18**(5):267-280. DOI: 10.1038/nrn.2017.26

[67] Brokaw EB, Lum PS, Cooper RA, Brewer BR. Using the kinect to limit abnormal kinematics and compensation strategies during therapy with end effector robots. In: Proceedings of the 2013 IEEE International Conference on Rehabilitation Robotics; 24-26 June; Seattle, WA, USA. 2013. DOI: 10.1109/ICORR.2013.6650384

[68] Da Gama A, Chaves T, Figueiredo L, Teichrieb V. Guidance and movement correction based on therapeutic movements for motor rehabilitation support systems. In: Proceedings of the 14th Symposium on Virtual and Augmented Reality; 28-31 May; Rio de Janeiro, Brazil. 2012. DOI: 10.1109/SVR.2012.15

[69] Nelson MJ, Crossley KM, Bourke MG, Russell TG. Telerehabilitation feasibility in total joint replacement. International Journal of Telerehabilitation. 2017;**9**(2):31-39. DOI: 10.5195/ijt.2017.6235

[70] Moffet H et al. In-home telerehabilitation compared with face-to-face rehabilitation after total knee arthroplasty: A noninferiority randomized controlled trial. The Journal of Bone & Joint Surgery. 2015;**97**(14):1129-1141. DOI: 10.2106/JBJS.N.01066

[71] Nelson M, Bourke M, Crossley K, Russell T. Telerehabilitation versus traditional care following total hip replacement: A randomized controlled trial protocol. JMIR Research Protocols. 2017;**6**(3):e34. DOI: 10.2196/resprot.7083

Chapter 3

A Systematic Review of Usability and Accessibility in Tele-Rehabilitation Systems

Jorge Luis Pérez Medina, Patricia Acosta-Vargas and Yves Rybarczyk

Abstract

The appropriate development of tele-rehabilitation platforms requires the involvement and iterative assessments of potential users and experts in usability. Usability consists of measuring the degree to which an interactive system can be used by specified final users to achieve quantified objectives with effectiveness, efficiency, and satisfaction in a quantified context of use. Usability studies need to be complemented by an accessibility assessment. Accessibility indicates how easy it is for a person to access any content, regardless of their physical, educational, social, psychological, or cultural conditions. This chapter intends to conduct a systematic review of the literature on usability and accessibility in tele-rehabilitation platforms carried out through the PRISMA method. To do so, we searched in ACM, IEEE Xplore, Google Scholar, and Scopus databases for the most relevant papers of the last decade. The main result of the usability shows that the user experience predominates over the heuristic studies, and the usability questionnaire most used in user experience is the SUS. The main result of the accessibility reveals that the topic is only marginally studied. In addition, it is observed that Web applications do not apply the physical and cognitive accessibility standards defined by the WCAG 2.1.

Keywords: usability, accessibility, telemedicine, tele-rehabilitation, systematic review

1. Introduction

Innovation and technological advances involve the offering of valuable products and services to improve the quality of life of citizens. In recent decades, the domain of telemedicine has reported advances in the control, monitoring and evaluation of various clinical conditions [1]. In the field of rehabilitation, numerous studies and state-of-the-arts from informatics perspective [2] and different areas of application [3, 4], show the effectiveness and advantages of the use of remote rehabilitation (or tele-rehabilitation) [5, 6]. Tele-rehabilitation aims to reduce the time and costs of offering rehabilitation services. The main objective is to improve the quality of life of patients [7]. Tele-rehabilitation cannot replace traditional neurological rehabilitation [8]. It is considered as a partial replacement of face-to-face physical rehabilitation [9]. Tele-rehabilitation uses mainly two groups of technologies: (1) wearable devices and (2) vision-based systems based on depth cameras and intelligent algorithms [10]. In [5], the authors describe and analyze some characteristics and typical requirements tele-rehabilitation systems.

Design and conception of tele-rehabilitations platforms that do not consider guidelines, metrics, patterns, principles, or practice success factors can affect the access to the service, the effectiveness, quality, and usefulness. It can cause problems of confusion, error, stress, and abandonment of the rehabilitation plan. Therefore, guaranteeing the correct use of these applications implies to incorporate different studies of usability in the life cycle of the interactive system. For this reason, aspects of human factors engineering in tele-rehabilitation systems have been studied with the aim of providing accessible, efficient, usable and understandable systems [11, 12].

User-centered agile development (UCD) approaches allows developers to specify and design the set of interfaces of any interactive system in a flexible and effective way [13, 14]. The agile development life cycle centered on user experience (UX-ADLC) allows iteratively evaluating system interfaces based on the results of the previous iteration. The evaluation also includes the errors and usability problems encountered [15]. Thus, usability studies are an essential aspect of technology development [16]. This is the reason why designers need to meet usability and user experience objectives while adhering to agile principles of software development. Formative and summative usability tests are methods of evaluating software products widely adopted in user-centered design (UCD) [15] and agile UX development lifecycle. Both approaches are frequently used in the development of software applications. Rapid formative usability should be carried out so as to fulfill UX goals while satisfying end users' needs. Formative usability is used as an iterative test-and-refine method performed in the early steps of a design process, in order to detect and fix usability problems [15]. Summative usability allows for assuring, in later phases of the design, the quality of the user experience (UX) for a software product in development. The focus is on short work periods (or iterations) where usability tests (formative and summative) must be contemplated. This means that quick formative usability tests should be carried out to fulfill UX goals [17].

The ISO 9241-11 standard [18] is a framework for understanding and applying the concept of usability to situations in which people use interactive systems and other types of systems (including built environments), products (including industrial and consumer products) and services (including technical and personal services). Likewise, the usability standard ISO 9241-11 facilitates the measurement of the use of a product with the aim of achieving specific objectives with effectiveness, efficiency and satisfaction in a context of specific use [18].

Usability can be studied through software evaluation methods widely accepted in user centered design (UCD) [15]. It can be formative or summative [8]. Formative usability consists of a set of iterative tests carried out in the early stages of the design process. The aim of the tests is to refine and improve the software product, as well as to detect and solve potential usability problems. As a complement, the summative usability allows to obtain an evaluation of the user experience (UX) for a software product in development. Formative usability facilitates decision making during the design and development of the product, while summative usability is useful when studying user experience (UX).

Tullis and Stetson [19] evaluated the effectiveness of the most used questionnaires to measure the summative usability. The authors found that the System Usability Scale (SUS) [20] and the IBM Computer System Usability Questionnaire (CSUQ) [21] are the most effective. SUS provides a quick way for measuring the usability through user experience. It consists of a 10-item questionnaire with 5-likert scale range from "Strong Agree" to "Strongly Disagree." The CSUQ focuses on three main aspects: (1) the utility, which refers to the opinion of users regarding the ease of use, the ease of learning, the speed to perform the operations, the efficiency in completing tasks and subjective feeling; (2) the quality of the information which studies the subjectivity of the user regarding the management of system errors, the clarity of the information and the intelligibility; and finally, (3) the quality of the interface which measures the affective component of the user's attitude in the use of the system.

Large part of the tasks in the tele-rehabilitation systems are carried out by patients who require to treat a temporary disability. Considering the special needs of these users, usability evaluations alone cannot guarantee an appropriate design of the system. On the contrary, accessibility studies can provide the mechanisms to offer the same means of use to all users of any interactive system. A study combining usability and accessibility was presented in [22]. The study analyzes how remote and/or video monitoring technologies affect the accessibility, effectiveness, quality and usefulness of the services offered by tele-rehabilitation systems. To do this, the authors provide an overview of the fundamentals necessary for the analysis of usability, in addition to analyzing the strengths and limitations of various tele-rehabilitation technologies, considering how technologies interact with the clinical needs of end users such as accessibility, effectiveness, quality and utility of the service [22].

For many people, the Web is a fundamental part of everyday life. Therefore, a fundamental aspect to ensure the inclusivity of a Website is its accessibility. For example, people who cannot use their arms to write on their computer can use a mouth pencil [23]. Or someone who cannot listen well can use subtitles to understand a video. Also, a person who has a low vision can use a screen reader to listen what is written on the screen [24]. Therefore, Web accessibility means that people with disabilities can use the Web without any type of barriers [24]. There are several standards related to accessibility that provide guidelines and recommendations [25]. Some of the most important, according to the International Organization for Standardization (ISO), are the following ones:

- ISO 9241: covers ergonomics of human-computer interaction.
- ISO 14915 (software ergonomics for multimedia user interfaces): multimedia controls and navigation structure.
- ISO CD 9241-151 (software ergonomics for World Wide Web user interfaces): designs of Web user interfaces.
- ISO TS 16071 (guidance on accessibility for human-computer interface): recommendations for the design of systems and software applications that allows a greater accessibility to computer systems for users with disabilities.
- ISO CD 9241-20: accessibility guideline for information communication, equipment and services.

The Web Accessibility Initiative (WAI) [26] from the World Wide Web Consortium (W3C) [27] develops Web Content Accessibility Guidelines (WCAG) [28] 2.0 (at present 2.1) that covers a wide range of recommendations for making Web contents more accessible. These guidelines were considered a standard in

2012, the ISO/IEC 40500. Complementary to these guidelines are the W3C User Agent Accessibility guidelines [29] (UAAG) and Authoring tool Accessibility guidelines [30] (ATAG), which addresses the current technological capabilities to modify the presentation based on the device capabilities and the preferences of the user.

The World Wide Web Consortium (W3C) provides international standards to make the Web as accessible as possible. It comprises the Web 2.0 Content Accessibility Guidelines (WCAG 2.0) [31], also known as the ISO 40500 [32], which are adapted to the European Standard called EN 301549 [33].

The current version of the accessibility guidelines is "Web Content Accessibility Guidelines 2.1" (WCAG 2.1) [23]. WCAG 2.1 consists of 4 principles, 13 guidelines and 76 compliance criteria. The four principles refer to [34].

Principle 1—perceptibility: refers to the good practices regarding the presentation of information and user interface components. It consists of 4 guidelines and 29 compliance criteria.

Principle 2—operability: the components of the user interface and navigation must be operable. It includes 5 guidelines and 29 compliance criteria.

Principle 3—comprehensibility: the information and user interface management must be understandable. It has 3 guidelines and 17 compliance criteria.

Principle 4—robustness: the content must be robust enough to rely on the interpretation of a wide variety of user agents, including assistive technologies. It includes a guideline and three compliance criteria.

Usability and accessibility can be combined to achieve the development of more accessible, efficient, equitable and universal tele-rehabilitation systems. This chapter presents a systematic literature review of summative and formative usability studies as well as accessibility studies in the context of tele-rehabilitation systems. The remaining of the manuscript is composed of four sections. Section 2 presents the method used to proceed with the systematic review. Section 3 is a description of the most relevant papers in usability applied to tele-rehabilitation. Section 4 describes the results regarding the accessibility. And Section 5 draws conclusions on the main findings of this literature review.

2. Materials and methods

Systematic reviews and meta-analyzes are increasingly crucial in the area of health care. In order to optimize meta-analysis reports, an international group developed in 1996 a guide called the QUOROM Statement (Quality Of Reporting Of Meta-analyses), which focused on information from Meta-analysis of a randomized controlled trial [35]. One reason for changing the name from QUOROM to PRISMA (Preferred Reporting Items for Systematic Reviews and Meta-Analyses) was the desire to encompass both systematic reviews and meta analyses.

To improve the literature revision processes Quorum evolved until arriving at the PRISMA[1] declaration that consists of a checklist of 27 elements and a diagram of four-phase flow that is applied in this study.[2] The PRISMA statement helps authors improving the reports of systematic reviews and meta-analyzes. It is used as a basis to inform systematic reviews of other types of research.

[1] http://www.prisma-statement.org/

[2] http://prisma-statement.org/prismastatement/flowdiagram.aspx

In order to study the current state of Web platforms for tele-rehabilitation of patients with motor disability, we undertook a systematic review of the literature following the procedures specified in PRISMA. Based on that study, we formulate the following research questions:

1. Which studies currently exist on usability in the development of Web platforms for patients who need to perform a tele-rehabilitation?

2. Which studies currently exist related to Web accessibility in the development of inclusive platforms for patients who require a tele-rehabilitation?

The bibliographic search of usability and accessibility in the context of tele-rehabilitation systems was conducted using the ACM, Google Scholar, IEEE Xplore, and Scopus databases. **Table 1** shows the search chains used for each digital library, in order to obtain as many relevant studies as possible. Concerning the usability and accessibility, we limited our research to publications from 1990 to 2019.

There are many studies related to Web accessibility. Therefore, to ensure that the search is manageable and focused on tele-rehabilitation, we defined some inclusion and exclusion criteria when selecting the articles, such as:

- If the studies had been published in more than one journal or in the proceedings of a conference, we chose the complete version, only.

- We excluded non-scientific conferences and journals and papers that are out of the scope of the review.

Digital Library	Usability search	Accessibility search
ACM	acmdlTitle:(usability heuristic evaluation) AND recordAbstract:(tele-rehabilitation) AND keywords.author.keyword:(usability heuristic evaluation)	acmdlTitle:(web accessibility) AND recordAbstract:(telerehabilitation) AND keywords.author.keyword:(web accessibility)
IEEE Xplore	(("Document Title":usability OR "Document Title":"heuristic evaluation" OR "Document Title":"user experience") OR ("Publication Title":usability OR "Publication Title":"heuristic evaluation" OR "Publication Title":"user experience")) AND ("Abstract":tele-rehabilitation) AND ("Author Keywords":usability OR "Author Keywords":"heuristic evaluation" OR "Author Keywords":"user experience")	(("Document Title": accessibility OR "Document Title":"web" OR Document Title":"web accessibility") OR ("Publication Title": web accessibility OR "Publication Title":telerehabilitation)) AND ("Abstract": tele-rehabilitation) AND ("Author Keywords":web accessibility OR "Author Keywords":telerehabilitation)
Google Scholar	intitle:usability OR "heuristic evaluation" OR "User experience" "tele rehabilitation"	intitle: accessibility OR "web" OR "tele rehabilitation"
Scopus	(SRCTITLE (usability OR "heuristic evaluation" OR "user experience") OR TITLE (usability OR "heuristic evaluation" OR "user experience")) AND ABS (tele-rehabilitation*) AND KEY (usability OR "heuristic evaluation" OR "user experience") AND (PUBYEAR > 1989)	(SRCTITLE (accessibility OR "web") OR TITLE (accessibility OR "web") AND ABS (tele-rehabilitation*) AND KEY (accessibility OR "web") AND (PUBYEAR > 1989)

Table 1.
Search strings used for the literature review.

Digital Library	Usability studies	Accessibility studies
IEEE Xplore	1	26
Google Scholar	229	29
Scopus	1	7
ACM	12	14
Total	**243**	**76**

Table 2.
The number of research studies identified.

After the search was completed, 243 results were obtained for usability, and 76 results were obtained for accessibility (**Table 2**). Then, the title and the abstract of these articles were analyzed to identify their relevance to the topic of usability and accessibility in tele-rehabilitation systems.

We use the Start LaPes[3] 2.3.4.2 tool to analyze the databases that meet the search criteria and Mendeley Desktop[4] 1.19.3 to manage all the bibliography, details and appointments. This tool helps in the selection process of the scientific articles in such a way that it allows us to eliminate the duplicate articles, to register/filter the accepted and rejected articles in order to obtain reports that are adequate during the meta-analysis process.

Then, in order to study the current state of usability and accessibility related to tele-rehabilitation systems, we conducted a systematic review of the literature based on the PRISMA procedure [36].

When carrying out the literature review, studies that did not meet the established search criteria or referred to another type of usability/accessibility context were discarded. The phases of the selection process according to the PRISMA-based literature review for both themes, usability and accessibility, are detailed in the next two sections.

3. Usability review

The phases of the selection process for the literature review of papers on usability applied to tele-rehabilitation systems are detailed in **Figure 1**.

The 26 papers that were selected for further analysis are listed in **Table 3**.

Usability studies have a significant impact on the quality of the development of e-health systems. The potential for e-health to improve healthcare is partially dependent on its ease of use [45]. A systematic review presented in 2016 indicates that from 40 telemedicine studies, only 7.5% are focused on evaluating the user experience of the patients [46]. Academics, technical studies and scientific communities or special groups [60] have been conducted to evaluate the usability in e-health systems. [49] propose a methodological framework to perform user experience analysis of e-health technologies for patients' engagements. It considers a set of self-report measurements such as mental workload [61], system usability [20] and negative emotional responses [62], in order to provide descriptive data about the user experience of patients. [45] present a systematic review to identify psychometrically tested questionnaires that measure the usability of e-health tools, and to appraise their generalizability, attribute coverage, and quality. The main usability attributes found during the revisions were: learnability, efficiency, and satisfaction.

[3] http://lapes.dc.ufscar.br/tools/start_tool

[4] https://www.mendeley.com/download-desktop/

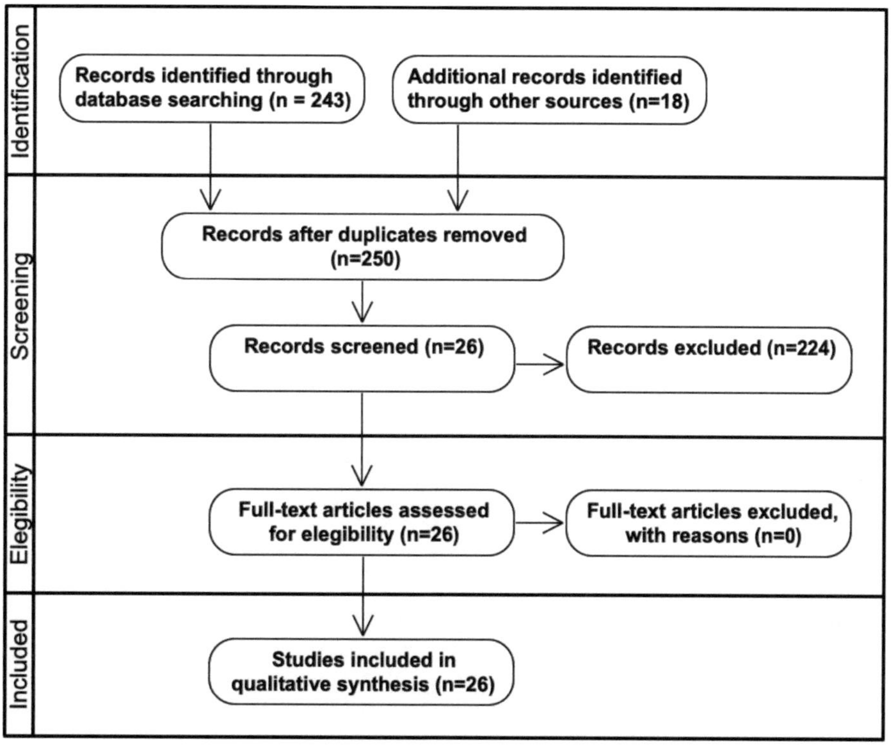

Figure 1.
PRISMA 2009 flow diagram chart that shows the selection process of the papers included in the literature review for usability.

Likewise, quality appraisal showed that face/content and construct validity were the most frequent types of validity assessed.

High levels of usability guarantee the substantial quality-of-life. This leads to the acceptance of tele-rehabilitation systems [58]. Likewise, a usability study, to evaluate patients' rehabilitation-evolution, is presented in [51] conclude that the usability is one of the advantages of the tele-rehabilitation system for both patients and professionals.

In [56], authors study the usability of a rehabilitation system designed to demonstrate, instruct and monitor a therapeutic exercise program. The evaluation of usability was carried out in two stages. The first stage consisted of a formative evaluation to identify initial usability problems, defects or omissions in the system. Secondly, user evaluation was conducted by using VRUSE, a computerized usability questionnaire explicitly designed for the evaluation of virtual reality applications [59].

Weiss et al. [55] present the development life cycle, including usability testing, of a low-cost remote rehabilitation system based on virtual reality technology. The solution was designed to provide remote rehabilitation of the upper extremities in patients who have had a stroke. The usability study was conducted with a population of eight patients. Usability was measured by the 5-point Short Feedback Questionnaire (SFQ) [57]. This instrument documents the enjoyment of participants and their perception of success and control while using the system. The perception was evaluated by using the Borg scale [63]. The subjective ratings were complemented by game performance scores.

In [54], a methodology for a home-based tele-rehabilitation system was presented. This work was done considering patients who require rehabilitation of the arms after having a stroke. The answers were collected via a series of structured

Title	Authors	Year
An Agile Approach to Improve the Usability of a Physical Telerehabilitation Platform	Pilco et al. [37]	2019
Usability study of a Web-Based Platform for Home Motor Rehabilitation	Pérez-Medina et al. [38]	2019
Implementation and Assessment of an Intelligent Motor Tele-Rehabilitation Platform	Rybarczyk, et al. [6]	2019
Analysis and Improvement of the Usability of a Tele-rehabilitation Platform for Hip Surgery Patients	Pilco et al. [39]	2018
A Telerehabilitation System for the Selection, Evaluation and Remote Management of Therapies	Anton et al. [40]	2018
Interaction with a Tele-Rehabilitation Platform Through a Natural User Interface: a Case Study of Hip Arthroplasty Patients	Rybarczyk et al. [41]	2018
Usability Evaluation of a Vibrotactile Feedback System in Stroke Subjects	Held et al. [42]	2017
On the Use of Natural User Interfaces in Physical Rehabilitation: a Web-based Application for Patients with Hip Prosthesis	Rybarczyk et al. [43]	2017
USEQ: A Short Questionnaire for Satisfaction Evaluation of Virtual Rehabilitation Systems	Gil-Gómez et al. [44]	2017
Towards usable E-health. A Systematic Review of Usability Questionnaires	Sousa et al. [45]	2017
A Renewed Framework for the Evaluation of Telemedicine	Jansen-Kosterink et al. [46]	2016
Development of the telehealth usability questionnaire (TUQ)	Parmanto et al. [47]	2016
Validation of a Kinect-based telerehabilitation system with total hip replacement patients	Anton et al. [48]	2016
Evaluating Patient Engagement and User Experience of a Positive Technology Intervention: The H-CIM Case	Triberti et al. [49]	2015
A novel knee rehabilitation system for the home	Ayoade et al. [50]	2014
Telerehabilitation web application for health care	Eguiluz-Perez et al. [51]	2014
SEQ: Suitability Evaluation Questionnaire for Virtual Rehabilitation Systems. Application in a Virtual Rehabilitation System for Balance Rehabilitation	Gil-Gómez et al. [52]	2013
Kires: a Kinect-based telerehabilitation system	Anton et al. [53]	2013
Assessment and training in home-based telerehabilitation of arm mobility impairment	Perry et al. [54]	2013
Development and validation of tele-health system for stroke rehabilitation	Weiss et al. [55]	2012
Usability evaluation of e-motion: a virtual rehabilitation system designed to demonstrate, instruct and monitor a therapeutic exercise program	Fitzgerald et al. [56]	2008
Short feedback questionnaire (SFQ) to enhance client-centered participation in virtual environments	Kizony et al. [57]	2006
Formative evaluation of a virtual reality telerehabilitation system for the lower extremity	Whitworth et al. [16]	2003
Dimensions of diversity in design of telerehabilitation systems for universal usability	Lathan et al. [58]	2000
VRUSE—a computerized diagnostic tool: for usability evaluation of virtual/synthetic environment systems	Kalawsky et al. [59]	1999
Evaluation—Methodology for Telematic Application Systems: Quality for Users and Context	Arnold et al. [60]	1997

Table 3.
List of the usability papers selected in this review.

interviews and seven point Likert-based evaluation questions measuring the level of agreement. Ayoade and Baillie [50] present the results of a randomized controlled study in which the authors investigated the usability and feasibility of a rehabilitation visualization system. This work has employed the principles of user-centered design throughout the development phases of the system. The study was performed with the SUS questionnaire [20]. Additionally, metrics significant for both patients and health professionals such as quality of life and the improved knee were studied.

Anton et al. [40] present a successful study of usability of a tele-rehabilitation system called KiReS [53]. The evaluation was made in a real scenario. The patients involved in the study underwent a total hip replacement surgery (THR). The study of the subjective perceptions of the patients when participating in the rehabilitation sessions was conducted through an empirical 5-point Likert scale questionnaire based on 13 statements and described in [48]. The instrument is structured in three sections: (1) the system, (2) the user experience, and (3) the user interface. The questionnaire also explores the prior knowledge that patients have regarding tele-rehabilitation systems. In general, the criticisms obtained by the patients were on the interfaces of the system [48].

In [16], the formative usability of the Rutgers Ankle Rehabilitation System (RARS) was studied involving three simultaneous users and a remote monitoring. The authors describe a usability evaluation process where engineers and physicians collaborated collaboratively. The usability study uses both traditional and empirical methods to assess the viability of the design of the interface.

A SUS questionnaire was used in order to study the usability and user acceptance of a sensor system called "Arm Usage Coach" (AUC) that provides VibroTactile (VT) feedback if the patient does not move the affected arm above a certain threshold level [42]. The study involved 10 patients who suffered a cardiovascular accident and had a mild to moderate arm impairment. The experiment made use of an AUC device on each wrist. VT feedback was given by the device on the affected arm. The usability was measured by using a semi-structured interview and also the SUS questionnaire. The results of the SUS questionnaire indicate that nine participants responded above 70% and one participant responded below 50%. It means that VT feedback is feasible and the AUC can be used as a tele-rehabilitation device to train and maintain upper extremity used in daily life tasks.

In [64], a web-based portal supporting several clinical activities and the Versatile Integrated System for Tele-rehabilitation video-conferencing system called VISYTER were evaluated through the IBM After-Scenario Questionnaire (ASQ) [65], the Post-Study System Usability Questionnaire (PSSUQ) [66], the Telehealth Usability Questionnaire (TUQ) [47], and two demographic surveys. The use of all these instruments allowed capturing subjective and objective information, resulting in an effective method to evaluate the usability in tele-rehabilitation systems.

The ePHoRt platform, which is a tele-rehabilitation system to support people recovering from a hip replacement surgery, has also been the subject of previous usability studies. The first reported usability study was conducted through the SUS. The overall score was 81 out of 100, which suggests a good usability of the Web application [43]. Next, in [39], the authors assert that the lack of usability may lead to problems of confusion, error, and delay, or even abandonment of the physical therapy. This study was a preliminary analysis based on an empirical heuristic evaluation. Unfortunately, the study was not significant enough since most of the interfaces evaluated do not represent the central aspects of the tele-rehabilitation system. Likewise, the study does not consider the efficiency, effectiveness, and satisfaction of patients. However, the authors suggest making successive evaluations of usability. So, a successive usability study was conducted and presented in [41]. The user experience was measured through two aspects: (1) the tasks completion time, and (2) the SUS questionnaire [20]. The results were correlated to an empirical sociodemographic questionnaire. The overall value of the SUS questionnaire was 76.1 out of 100, which can be considered an acceptable evaluation of the usability of the platform.

A more recent work conducted on an updated version of ePHoRt synthesizes the results obtained from a study of effectiveness, efficiency, and subjective user satisfaction [38]. Thirty nine participants tested the platform and were asked to evaluate its usability by using the IBM CSUQ. The empirical results based on subjective perception and self-reported feedback show that the application is useful, effective, efficient, easy to use, and its interfaces are acceptable. In addition, the evaluation of the user experience enables us to identify usability aspects that should be implemented, in order to improve the visual interface. The experiment indicates that user guidance is a critical aspect to ensure good usability of the tele-rehabilitation platform. Likewise, the error messages received by users should be as detailed as possible. Finally, in [6] the authors suggest to carry out usability tests with real patients and during the whole completion period of the rehabilitation program, as indicated in [36]. For this purpose, there are usability instruments specifically designed to measure the user experience with e-Health platforms, such as SEQ [52], USEQ [44] and TUQ [47].

Pilco et al. [37] is a very recent usability study that makes use of an agile user centered design process [13, 14] to assess the ePHoRt platform. The evaluation process stated with a heuristic evaluation by using the Nielsen's 10 heuristics principles [67]. In addition, a cognitive workload assessment was performed to complete the usability evaluation. Likewise, users were involved through all the stages of the iterative refinement process. Usability issues were progressively reduced by applying improvements suggested from the iterative assessments. For instance, usability issues originally cataloged as catastrophic were reduced to zero, major usability problems were diminished to 10 (2.75%), and minor usability problems were decreased to 141 (38.74%).

4. Accessibility review

The goal of most studies in the area of Web accessibility is to develop inclusive applications. However, this is a great challenge, because most applications do not follow the WCAG 2.1 standards suggested by the World Wide Web Consortium. Web accessibility studies have a high impact and significant benefits in the development of tele-rehabilitation applications. The World Health Organization (WHO) [68] estimates that more than 1 billion people live with some form of disability. This corresponds to approximately 15% of the world's population. Between 110 (2.2) and 190 million (3.8%) people aged 15 years and over have significant operational difficulties.

In addition, disability rates are growing because of the population aging and the chronic diseases associated with the increasing life expectation. Disability is now considered a human rights issue. People are disabled by society, not just by their bodies. Therefore, the universal access to technology must be considered in building an egalitarian society. After applying the search strings defined in **Table 1** and using the PRISMA method, a total of 76 publications were recorded for Web accessibility. In the screening phase, 14 duplicate articles were excluded, 11 articles meeting the inclusion parameters were included, and 51 were rejected as being out of the inclusion criteria. In the eligibility phase, a total of 11 articles were assessed as fully meeting the inclusion criteria (**Table 4**). The phases of the selection process according to the PRISMA literature review method are detailed in **Figure 2**.

Table 4 presents the references of the 11 articles selected in the literature review.

Calle-Jiménez et al. [69] explain some of the challenges that exist to develop accessible Web platforms in tele-rehabilitation applications for patients after a partial or total hip replacement, known as arthroplasty. The authors propose an iterative method to improve the level of accessibility through automatic evaluation tools. Three online WAVE, AChecker, and TAW tools were applied in the study. The

Title	Authors	Year
Analysis and improvement of the web accessibility of a tele-rehabilitation platform for hip arthroplasty patients	Calle-Jimenez et al. [69]	2019
Educational resources accessible on the tele-rehabilitation platform	Acosta-Vargas et al. [70]	2019
An mHealth App for Users with Dexterity Impairments: Accessibility Study	Yu et al. [71]	2019
Towards Web Accessibility in Tele-rehabilitation Platforms	Acosta-Vargas et al. [72]	2018
Personalized technology-enhanced training for people with cognitive impairment	Buzzi et al. [73]	2018
Design and Development of One-Switch Video Games for Children with Severe Motor Disabilities	López et al. [74]	2017
Internet Use By People Living With Neurological Conditions: a Scoping Study	Siegert et al. [75]	2015
Computer-based cognitive training in adults with Down's syndrome	Bargagna et al. [76]	2014
Visual Complexity, Player Experience, Performance and Physical Exertion in Motion-based Games for Older Adults	Smeddinck et al. [77]	2013
Tele-rehabilitation interface strategies for enhancing access to health services for persons with diverse abilities and preferences	Winters [78]	2013
Accessibility of e-health services for people with disabilities	Bąkała et al. [79]	2010

Table 4.
Summary of the accessibility papers selected in this review.

results of the analysis indicate that the studied platform does not comply with all WCAG 2.0 accessibility standards.

Acosta-Vargas et al. [70] propose to apply the Accessibility Guidelines for educational content, in accordance with the Web Accessibility Initiative, to a tele-rehabilitation platform. The accessibility of the Web resources is assessed by using the Photosensitive Epilepsy Analysis Tool (PEAT). This open access software application applies several WCAG 2.0 standards and is combined with a manual evaluation method. The results of the study show that the multimedia resources evaluated do not reach an acceptable level of accessibility, as well.

Yu et al. [71] present a mobile health system (m-Health) to assist people with chronic diseases and disabilities in their self-management regimens. The authors studied the accessibility by using the WCAG 1.0 and 2.0 guidelines. The evaluation process was performed manually. The results indicate that on the importance of customization of interfaces to improve accessibility.

Acosta-Vargas et al. [72] present an accessibility study performed on a Web platform to promote a physical rehabilitation of patients with an arthroplasty. Web Content Accessibility Guidelines (WCAG) 2.0 and Website Accessibility Conformance Evaluation Methodology (WCAG-EM) 1.0 were applied. The authors used tools through plugins installed in the Web browser. WAVE,[5] Siteimprove,[6] Open WAX,[7] and Tenon[8] were used. The results indicate that the tele-rehabilitation platform requires improvements to reach an appropriate level of Web accessibility.

[5] https://wave.webaim.org/

[6] https://siteimprove.com/

[7] https://github.com/goonoo/OpenWAX

[8] http://tenon.io/

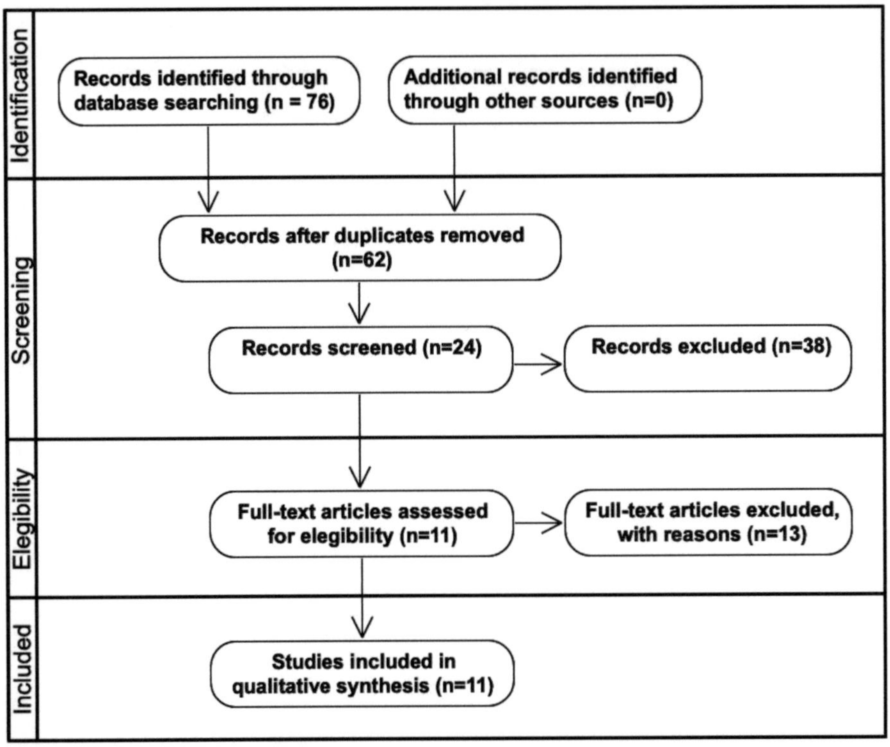

Figure 2.
PRISMA 2009 flow diagram chart showing the selection process.

Buzzi et al. [73] propose a Web platform to offer accessible games to individuals with cognitive disabilities, such as people with Down Syndrome (DS). Some WCAG 2.0 guidelines are applied manually, but no tools are applied in accessibility evaluation. The results of this study highlight the importance of motivation and flexibility to personalize the content according to the limitations of each user. Based on this experience, some basic guidelines for refining protocols for accessibility testing with people with DS have been proposed to maximize engagement, increase usability, and gather feedback to improve the accessibility of game design.

López et al. [74] argue that video games are not played just for fun, but are a useful tool for children's cognitive, emotional and social development. The article contributes to reducing accessibility barriers. The development game, called "Gaming NOMON" or (GNomon) is based on a guide of accessibility for videogames. It application has been evaluated for children with severe motor disabilities, so the study can serve as lessons learned for future research and design of accessible video games.

Richard Siegert et al. [75] indicate that little is known about Internet use among people with disabilities. This study explores how people with neurological conditions, such as multiple sclerosis, traumatic brain injury, or stroke use the new technologies. Some WCAG standards were applied in the research. The authors are not concerned with evaluating the accessibility per se. but the potential benefits of Internet for health and the well-being of people with disabilities.

Also, Bargagna et al. [76] describe a set of computerized exercises designed for cognitive training of adults with Down Syndrome. The objective of the study is to develop a tele-rehabilitation platform by following WCAG 2.0 guidelines for Web application. For future studies, the researchers propose to develop more training games to investigate the long-term effects of software use and assess its relevance in preserving cognitive capacity and individual autonomy in everyday activities.

Smeddinck et al. [77] point out that motion-based video games may have a variety of benefits for players and are increasingly applied in physiotherapy, rehabilitation, and prevention of older adults. The authors suggest that aspects of accessibility and immersion should be considered if the potential benefits of motion-based video games are to be harnessed for target groups with a broad spectrum of visual impairments. The application does not use WCAG-related guidelines, and does not apply specific tools to assess Web accessibility. The results show that visual complexity affects the perception of the games. The findings of this study can help to improve the design of motion-based games for therapy and rehabilitation in older adults.

Winters [78] proposes a preliminary classification scheme for tele-rehabilitation processes in order to apply it to human factors and to the analysis of the accessibility of electronic systems. The study proposes a novel framework in the development of interfaces that lead to a universal access to tele-rehabilitation for people with disabilities. This study makes use of some guidelines related to WCAG and Section 508. The results suggest that during the development of Web applications, accessibility guidelines should be considered in order to have more inclusive Websites.

Finally, Bąkała et al. [79] explain the concept of online health services in Poland, which tends to include people with disabilities. The researchers present a comparative analysis of e-health solutions in Poland and in other European countries. They conclude that there are possibilities to adapt existing services, in order to include people with disabilities. The study analyses the WCAG guidelines, but it does not apply tools to evaluate tele-rehabilitation platforms.

5. Conclusions

The main result of the usability review for tele-rehabilitation systems shows that the user experience predominates over the heuristic studies, and the most used questionnaire to assess user experience is the SUS. Even though it would be relevant to carry out user experiences with real patients and in real conditions, there are still few usability questionnaires proposed in tele-rehabilitation. Likewise, studies do not measure the performance of the patients in terms of completion time of the tasks and percentage of errors during the rehabilitation exercises.

Regarding the question of Web accessibility in tele-rehabilitation platforms, the review shows that this topic is still marginally studied. Many applications do not care about developing accessible and inclusive platforms. Some studies refer to Section 508 and WCAG 1.0 and 2.0 guidelines, but they are not applied in their entirety in addition, no work applies the WCAG 2.1, which is the most recent Web accessibility guideline. It is also to mention the fact that the analyzed studies lack the application of combined methods to ensure an adequate level of Web accessibility. Thus, our review suggests that the development of future e-Health applications should apply the guidelines of WCAG 2.1 that will allow access to all types of users regardless of their physical and cognitive abilities. This conclusion is particularly relevant in the case of the development of tele-rehabilitation platforms, which should include both usability and accessibility iterative tests.

Author details

Jorge Luis Pérez Medina*, Patricia Acosta-Vargas and Yves Rybarczyk
Intelligent and Interactive Systems Lab (SI2 Lab), Universidad de Las Américas (UDLA), Quito, Ecuador

*Address all correspondence to: jorge.perez.medina@udla.edu.ec

References

[1] Flodgren G, Rachas A, Farmer A, Inzitari M, Shepperd S. Interactive telemedicine: Effects on professional practice and health care outcomes. 2015

[2] Parmanto B, Saptono A. Telerehabilitation: State-of-the-art from an informatics perspective. International Journal of Telerehabilitation. 2009;**1**(1):73-84

[3] Peretti A, Amenta F, Tayebati SK, Nittari G, Mahdi SS. Telerehabilitation: Review of the state-of-the-art and areas of application. JMIR Rehabilitation and Assistive Technologies. 2017;**4**(2):e7

[4] Rogante M, Grigioni M, Cordella D, Giacomozzi C. Ten years of telerehabilitation: A literature overview of technologies and clinical applications. NeuroRehabilitation. 2010;**27**(4):287-304

[5] Rybarczyk Y, Kleine Deters J, Cointe C, Esparza D. Smart web-based platform to support physical rehabilitation. Sensors. 2018;**18**(5):1344

[6] Rybarczyk Y et al. Implementation and assessment of an intelligent motor tele-rehabilitation platform. Electronics. 2019;**8**(1):58

[7] McCue M, Fairman A, Pramuka M. Enhancing quality of life through telerehabilitation. Physical Medicine and Rehabilitation Clinics of North America. 2010;**21**(1):195-205

[8] Rollnik JD, Pohl M, Mokrusch T, Wallesch CW. Telerehabilitation kann die klassische neurologische rehabilitation nicht ersetzen. Nervenarzt. 2017;**88**(10):1192-1193

[9] Jansen-Kosterink S, in't Veld RH, Hermens H, Vollenbroek-Hutten M. A telemedicine service as partial replacement of face-to-face physical rehabilitation: The relevance of use. Telemedicine and e-Health. 2015;**21**(10):808-813

[10] Barriga A, Conejero J, Hernández J, Jurado E, Moguel E, Sánchez-Figueroa F. A vision-based approach for building telecare and telerehabilitation services. Sensors. 2016;**16**(10):1724

[11] Lathan CE, Kinsella A, Rosen MJ, Winters J, Trepagnier C. Aspects of human factors engineering in home telemedicine and telerehabilitation systems. Telemedicine Journal. 1999;**5**(2):169-175

[12] Brennan DM, Barker LM. Human factors in the development and implementation of telerehabilitation systems. Journal of Telemedicine and Telecare. 2008;**14**(2):55-58

[13] Pérez-Medina JL, Vanderdonckt J. A tool for multi-surface collaborative sketching. In: WorkShop Cross-Surface 2016: Third International Workshop on Interacting with Multi-Device Ecologies "in the wild". 2016

[14] Pérez-Medina JL, Vanderdonckt J. Sketching by cross-surface collaboration. In: Rocha Á. PM, Ferrás C, editors. Information Technology and Systems., Advances. Cham: Springer; 2019. pp. 386-397

[15] Kieffer S, Ghouti A, Macq B. The agile ux development lifecycle: Combining formative usability and agile methods. 2017

[16] Whitworth E, Lewis JA, Boian R, Tremaine M, Burdea G, Deutsch JE. Formative evaluation of a virtual reality telerehabilitation system for the lower extremity. In: Proceedings of the 2nd International Workshop on Virtual Rehabilitation (IWVR2003); Piscataway, NJ, USA. 2003. pp. 21-22

[17] Sy D. Adapting usability investigations for agile user-centered design. Journal of usability Studies. 2007;**2**:112-132

[18] Stewart T. Ergonomic requirements for office work with visual display terminals (VDTs): Part 11: Guidance on usability. International Organization for Standardization (ISO). 1998;**9241**:3-8

[19] Tullis TS, Stetson JN. A comparison of questionnaires for assessing website usability. In: Usability Professional Association Conference. Vol. 1. 2004

[20] Brooke J et al. SUS-A quick and dirty usability scale. Usability Evaluation In Industry. 1996;**189**(194):4-7

[21] Lewis JR. IBM computer usability satisfaction questionnaires: Psychometric evaluation and instructions for use. International Journal of Human Computer Interaction. 1995;**7**(1):57-78

[22] Pramuka M, van Roosmalen L. Telerehabilitation technologies: Accessibility and usability. International Journal of Telerehabilitation. 2009;**1**(1):85-98

[23] World Wide Web Consortium (W3C), Web Content Accessibility Guidelines (WCAG) 2.1. 2018

[24] World Wide Web Consortium (W3C). WCAG 2.1 is a W3C Recommendation|W3C Blog. 2018

[25] Bevan N. International Standards for HCI and Usability. International Journal of Human-Computer Studies. 2001;**55**(4):533-552

[26] World Wide Web Consortium (W3C). Web Accessibility Initiative. 2017

[27] W3C. Web Content Accessibility Guidelines (WCAG) 2.0[Online]. Available from: https://www.w3.org/TR/2008/REC-WCAG20-20081211/ [Accessed: 05-Jan-2019]

[28] World Wide Web Consortium (W3C). Web Content Accessibility Guidelines 2.0. 2008

[29] W3C. User Agent Accessibility Guidelines (UAAG) Overview | Web Accessibility Initiative (WAI) | W3C [Online]. Available from: https://www.w3.org/WAI/standards-guidelines/uaag/ [Accessed: 05-Jan-2019]

[30] W3C. Authoring Tool Accessibility Guidelines (ATAG) Overview | Web Accessibility Initiative (WAI) [Online]. Available from: https://www.w3.org/WAI/standards-guidelines/atag/ [Accessed: 05-Jan-2019]

[31] World Wide Web Consortium (W3C). Web Content Accessibility Guidelines (WCAG) 2.0. 2018

[32] ISO/IEC. 40500:2012 Information technology—W3C Web Content Accessibility Guidelines (WCAG) 2.0. 2012

[33] ESTI. EN 301 549 v2.1.2 (2018-08). Vol. 1. 2014. pp. 1-138

[34] World Wide Web Consortium (W3C). Introduction to Web Accessibility|Web Accessibility Initiative (WAI)|W3C [Online]. Available from: https://www.w3.org/WAI/fundamentals/accessibility-intro/#context [Accessed: 19-Nov-2018]

[35] Moher D, Liberati A, Tetzlaff J, Altman DG, Prisma Group. Preferred reporting items for systematic reviews and meta-analyses: The PRISMA statement (reprinted from annals of internal medicine). Annals of Internal Medicine. 2009;**151**(4):264-269

[36] Liberati A et al. The PRISMA statement for reporting systematic reviews and meta-analyses of studies

that evaluate health care interventions: Explanation and elaboration. PLoS Medicine. 2009;**6**(7):e1000100

[37] Pilco H et al. An agile approach to improve the usability of a physical telerehabilitation platform. Applied Sciences. 2019;**9**(3):480

[38] Pérez-Medina JL et al. Usability study of a web-based platform for home motor rehabilitation. IEEE Access. 2019;**7**:7932-7947

[39] Pilco H et al. Analysis and improvement of the usability of a tele-rehabilitation platform for hip surgery patients. In: International Conference on Applied Human Factors and Ergonomics. 2018. pp. 197-209

[40] Anton D, Berges I, Bermúdez J, Goñi A, Illarramendi A. A telerehabilitation system for the selection, evaluation and remote management of therapies. Sensors. 2018;**18**(5):1459

[41] Rybarczyk Y et al. Interaction with a tele-rehabilitation platform through a natural user interface: A case study of hip arthroplasty patients. In: International Conference on Applied Human Factors and Ergonomics; 2018. pp. 246-256

[42] Held JP, Klaassen B, van Beijnum B-JF, Luft AR, Veltink PH. Usability evaluation of a vibrotactile feedback system in stroke subjects. Frontiers in Bioengineering and Biotechnology. 2017;**4**:98

[43] Rybarczyk Y et al. On the use of natural user interfaces in physical rehabilitation: A web-based application for patients with hip prosthesis. Journal of Science and Technology of the Arts. 2018;**10**(2):2

[44] Gil-Gómez J-A, Manzano-Hernández P, Albiol-Pérez S, Aula-Valero C, Gil-Gómez H, Lozano-Quilis J-A. USEQ: A short questionnaire for satisfaction evaluation of virtual rehabilitation systems. Sensors. 2017;**17**(7):1589

[45] Sousa VEC, Lopez KD. Towards usable e-health. Applied clinical informatics. 2017;**8**(02):470-490

[46] Jansen-Kosterink S, Vollenbroek-Hutten M, Hermens H. A renewed framework for the evaluation of telemedicine. In: Venice, Italy: 8th International Conference on eHealth, Telemedicine, and Social Medicine: eTELEMED. Vol. 2016. 2016

[47] Parmanto B, Lewis AN, Graham KM, Bertolet MH. Development of the telehealth usability questionnaire (TUQ). International Journal of Telerehabilitation. 2016;**8**(1):3-10

[48] Anton D, Nelson M, Russell T, Goñi A, Illarramendi A. Validation of a Kinect-based telerehabilitation system with total hip replacement patients. Journal of Telemedicine and Telecare. 2016;**22**(3):192-197

[49] Triberti S, Barello S, Graffigna G, Riva G, Candelieri A, Archetti F. Evaluating patient engagement and user experience of a positive technology intervention: The H-CIM case. In: Patient Engagement. A Consumer-Centered Model to Innovate Healthcare. Sciendo Migration: Walter de Gruyter GmbH; 2015. pp. 66-77. DOI: 10.1515/9783110452440-007

[50] Ayoade M, Baillie L. A novel knee rehabilitation system for the home. In: Proceedings of the SIGCHI Conference on Human Factors in Computing Systems (CHI '14). New York, NY, USA: ACM; 2014. pp. 2521-2530. DOI: 10.1145/2556288.2557353

[51] Eguiluz-Perez G, Garcia-Zapirain B. Telerehabilitation web application for health care professionals and adults with multiple sclerosis. In: Proceedings of the 8th International Conference on Pervasive Computing Technologies for Healthcare. 2014. pp. 286-289

[52] Gil-Gómez J-A, Gil-Gómez H, Lozano-Quilis J-A, Manzano-Hernández P, Albiol-Pérez S, Aula-Valero C. SEQ: Suitability evaluation questionnaire for virtual rehabilitation systems. Application in a virtual rehabilitation system for balance rehabilitation. In: Proceedings of the 7th International Conference on Pervasive Computing Technologies for Healthcare; 2013. pp. 335-338

[53] Antón D, Goñi A, Illarramendi A, Torres-Unda JJ, Seco J. KiReS: A Kinect-based telerehabilitation system. In: EEE 15th International Conference on e-Health Networking, Applications and Services (Healthcom). Lisbon, Portugal: IEEE, Piscataway, NJ; 2013. pp. 444-448

[54] Perry JC, Rodriguez-de-Pablo C, Cavallaro FI, Belloso A, Keller T. Assessment and training in home-based telerehabilitation of arm mobility impairment. Journal of Accessibility and Design for All. 2013;**3**(2):44-75

[55] Weiss PL et al. Development and validation of tele-health system for stroke rehabilitation. In: Proceedings of the 9th International Conference on Disability, Virtual Reality and Associated Technologies (ICDVRAT); 0-12 Sept. 2012; Laval, France. pp. 33-40. ISBN 978-0-7049-1545-9

[56] Fitzgerald D, Kelly D, Ward T, Markham C, Caulfield B. Usability evaluation of e-motion: A virtual rehabilitation system designed to demonstrate, instruct and monitor a therapeutic exercise programme. In: Virtual Rehabilitation; IEEE. 2008. pp. 144-149

[57] Kizony R, Katz N, Rand D, Weiss PLT. Short feedback questionnaire (SFQ) to enhance client-centered participation in virtual environments. Cyberpsychology & Behavior. 2006;**9**(6):687-688

[58] Lathan G. Dimensions of diversity in design of telerehabilitation systems for universal usability. In: John Thomas, editor. Proceedings on the 2000 Conference on Universal Usability (CUU '00). New York, NY, USA: ACM; 2000. pp. 61-62. DOI: 10.1145/355460.355473

[59] Kalawsky RS. VRUSE{−} a computerised diagnostic tool: For usability evaluation of virtual/ synthetic environment systems. Applied Ergonomics. 1999;**30**(1):11-25

[60] Arnold AG, van den Anker FWG. Evaluation methodology telematics systems: Quality for users and context, a CHI 97 special interest group. SIGCHI Bulletin. 1997;**29**(4). Available from: https://homepages.cwi.nl/~steven/sigchi/bulletin/1997.4/arnold.html

[61] Hart SG, Staveland LE. Development of NASA-TLX (task load index): Results of empirical and theoretical research. Advances in Psychology. 1988;**52**:139-183

[62] Spielberger CD. Manual for the State-Trait Anxiety Inventory STAI (Form Y) ('Self-Evaluation Questionnaire'. 1983

[63] Borg G. Psychophysical scaling with applications in physical work and the perception of exertion. Scandinavian Journal of Work, Environment & Health. 1990;**16**(suppl. 1):55-58

[64] Schutte J, Gales S, Filippone A, Saptono A, Parmanto B, McCue M. Evaluation of a telerehabilitation system for community-based rehabilitation. International Journal of Telerehabilitation. 2012;**4**(1):15-24

[65] Lewis JR, R J. Psychometric evaluation of an after-scenario questionnaire for computer usability studies. ACM SIGCHI Bulletin. 1990;**23**(1):78-81

[66] Lewis JR. Psychometric evaluation of the post-study system usability questionnaire: The

PSSUQ. Proceedings of the Human Factors and Ergonomics Society. Annual Meeting. Human Factors and Ergonomics Society. Annual Meeting. 1992;**36**(16):1259-1260

[67] Jakob NJ. Usability inspection methods. In: Plaisant C, editor. Conference Companion on Human Factors in Computing Systems (CHI '94). New York, NY, USA: ACM; 1994. pp. 413-414. DOI: 10.1145/259963.260531

[68] World Health Organization (WHO). Disability and health. 2018

[69] Calle-Jimenez T et al. Analysis and improvement of the web accessibility of a tele-rehabilitation platform for hip arthroplasty patients. In: AHFE International Conference on Human Factors and Systems Interaction; 2018; Vol. 781. Escuela Politécnica Nacional, Quito, Ecuador: Springer Verlag; 2019. pp. 233-245

[70] Acosta-Vargas P et al. Educational resources accessible on the tele-rehabilitation platform. In: Nunes I, editor. Advances in Human Factors and Systems Interaction. AHFE 2018. Advances in Intelligent Systems and Computing. Cham: Springer; 2018. Vol. 781. pp. 210-220

[71] Yu D, Parmanto B, Dicianno B. An mHealth app for users with dexterity impairments: Accessibility study. JMIR mHealth uHealth. 2019;7(1):e202

[72] Acosta-vargas P, Rybarczyk Y, Pérez J, González M, Jimenes K, Leconte L. Towards web accessibility in telerehabilitation platforms. In: ETCM; 2018

[73] Buzzi MC, Buzzi M, Perrone E, Senette C. Personalized technology-enhanced training for people with cognitive impairment. Universal Access in the Information Society. 2018;**0**(0):1-17

[74] López SA, Corno F, De Russis L. Design and development of one-switch video games for children with severe motor disabilities. ACM Transactions on Accessible Computing. 2017;**10**(4):1-42

[75] Richard Siegert CF, Snell D, Sullivan M, Babbage D. Internet use by people living with neurological conditions: A scoping study. 2015

[76] Bargagna S, Bozza M, Buzzi MC, Buzzi M, Doccini E, Perrone E. Computer-based cognitive training in adults with Down's syndrome. In: 8th International Conference on Universal Access in Human-Computer Interaction, UAHCI 2014—Held as Part of 16th International Conference on Human-Computer Interaction, HCI International 2014; Vol. 8514 LNCS, no. PART 2. 2014. IRCCS Stella Maris, viale del Tirreno 331, 56128 Calambrone (PI), Italy: Springer Verlag; 2014. pp. 197-208

[77] Smeddinck J, Gerling KM, Tiemkeo S. Visual complexity, player experience, performance and physical exertion in motion-based games for older adults. In: Proc. 15th Int. ACM SIGACCESS Conf. Comput. Access.—ASSETS'13. 2013. pp. 1-8

[78] Winters JM. Telerehabilitation interface strategies for enhancing access to health services for persons with diverse abilities and preferences. In: In Telerehabilitation. London:Springer; 2013. pp. 57-78

[79] Bąkała A, Korczak K. "Accessibility of e-health services for people with disabilities," Pr. Nauk. Uniw. Ekon. we Wrocławiu. Informatyka Ekonomiczna. 2010;**18**:31-30

Chapter 4

Dual Loop Theory: Eidetic Feedback Control and Predictive Feedback Control

Keiko Tsujioka

Abstract

We have been studying on human information processing and finding out two types of feedback loop, positive and negative which are used when people understand a sentence. Former one is eidetic feedback control by visual sensory organs with encoding short-term memory (STM). Latter one is predictive feedback control by phonological imagery and schema, which help recall and reconstruction or reformation of concepts concerning with long term memory (LTM). Moreover, those strategies might be related to their behavior or attitudes. We have hypotheses that there are individual differences depending on strategies how two loops are used. Those findings must lead coordinating transformation and learning control for AI doctor or care assistive robots, which are required to interact with various types of people so that they can predict their behavior and attitudes through feedforward control.

Keywords: dual loop theory, eidetic feedback control, predictive feedback control, human information processing, human-machine interaction

1. Introduction

It has been becoming a key factor for artificial intelligent computers, which are composed of modern style machine learning system, how they are able to get involved with human.

Then, in our study, we have conducted experiments over a decade so that we can clarify human information processing, aiming to improve their interaction of AI doctor or support robot with human being by predicting their behavior from finding out their individual cognitive traits [1].

Specifically, we have predicted that their traits concerning with information processing would become clearer by comparing response time to short sentences between presenting with sound voice and letters. Those short sentences which are 120 questionnaires of psychological testing (YGPI) ask subjects whether they are the same or not, comparing with their daily ordinary behavior [2]. In other words, those questionnaires are concerning autobiographical memory [3], which are not effects of their knowledge or academic ability, but personality of 12 factors which divided into two factors, emotional and non-emotional [4–6].

From the results of our previous study, correlation coefficient between individual response time and the criteria of measurement (duration of each reading questions or the number of words in one question) in the experiment by sound voice (listening) was higher than those of by letters (silent reading). And more, there was greater dispersion of response time among subjects in presenting letters experiment than former ones. From these reasons, we predicted that there would be differentiation of individual traits of information processing for letters than those of sound voice [6, 7].

We have therefore examined response time by silent reading individually and found out that there were persons of Visual type (N = 12 of 98, $r < 0.3$) whose correlation coefficients were much lower than those of Auditory type (N = 31 of 98, $r > 0.5$). In addition to this, the average of response time of Visual type persons was significantly shorter than those of Auditory type [6, 7].

Moreover, we have inspected reaction time of silent reading, especially among Intermediate type (N = 55), and found out there were another pattern of information processing between Emotional and non-Emotional questionnaires [6, 7].

In this paper, we have categorized two types, Eidetic type and Adjusting type, whose correlation coefficients and response time patters were different with each other. From these viewpoints, we had formulated a hypothesis (dual loop theory) and verified them by the experiments of practical collaborative learning in nursing class. One loop might be concerning positive feedback control (PFC) and other one might be negative feedback control (NFC) [8, 9]. Epidemic type persons might have tendency of PFC while they are solving problems. On the other hand, Adjustive type might tend coordinating two cycles (PFC and NFC) [10, 11]. We had revealed differentiations between the two types of behaviors.

Consequently, we would like to propose that the results of this study might help AI computer to learn machinery, thereby analyzing Big Data of various students' results and predicting their individual pattern of behavior so that it can support for personalized education, for instance, optimizing combination for collaborative learning.

2. Methods

2.1 System

Our purpose of this study is to clarify human information processing in order to optimize machine learning for AI computer, which is intended to communicate interactively with human being.

At first, there were problems in collaborative learning of practical nursing class at university and we needed to find the solution. After investigating them in 2014, we have found that there was the main cause of those problems which were failing at a relationship among team members. Then, we have developed the Personalized Education and Learning Support System (PELS) in 2015 [1], which helps instructors and learners to work interactively with each other by optimizing combinations of team members from the viewpoint of personality (**Figure 1**).

The main system of PELS is Big Data processing system (1) (**Figure 2**), [11], which gathers students' various data, for instance. measuring their traits (2), recording their behavior, results of their performance, questionnaires, and so on, and analyzes them (3), then inform them to instructors (4) so that they can make plans for instructions included teaming members for collaborative learning interactively.

The result of students' performances at the first semester (**Figure 3**, upper) has been improving after introducing PELS to nursing classes, comparing the average scores with the conventional form in 2014; on the other hand, it has been dealing from 2015 to 2017 at second semester (**Figure 3**, right). We have supposed that the

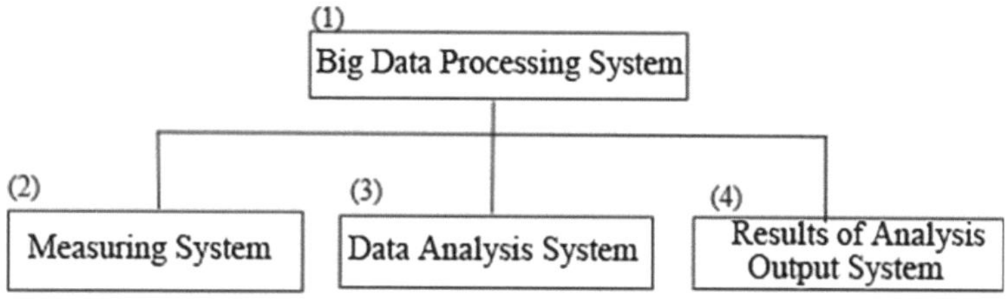

Figure 1.
Local search for solution of combinatorial optimization.

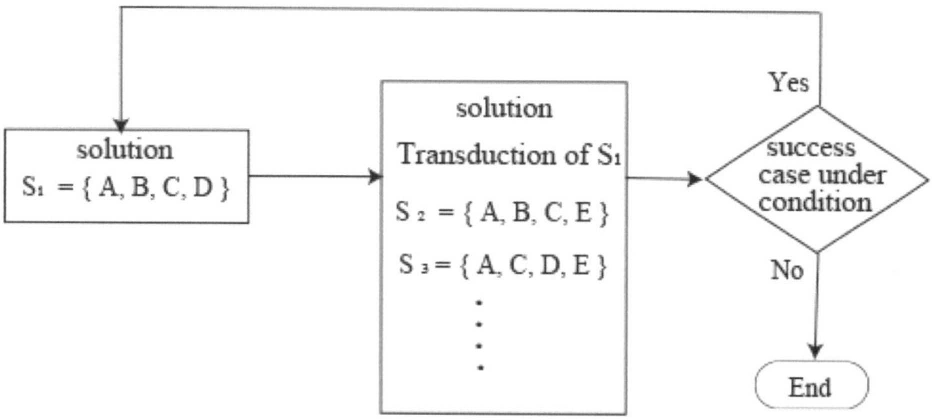

Figure 2.
Local search for solution of combinatorial optimization.

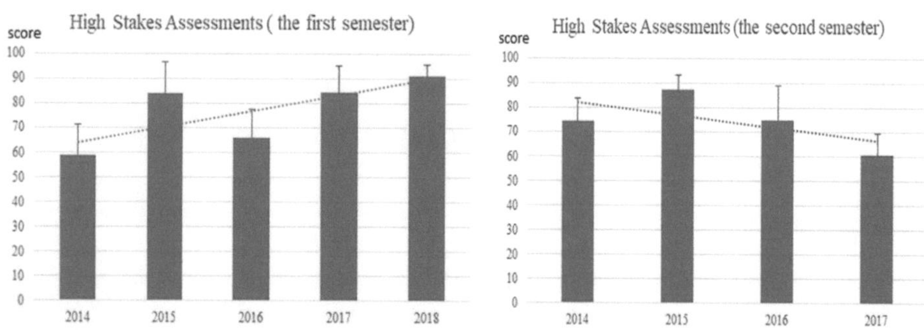

Figure 3.
Changing scores over the years.

reason of those phenomena might be influenced by not only their personality but also their cognitive traits [12], especially concerning with language information processing, because our lifestyle has been changed dramatically in digital society even in educational field [6, 7].

From these reasons, we have been examining PELS from the viewpoints of optimizing combination for teaming members, through comparing performances and individual differences between successful and unsuccessful teams. Combinatorial optimization, however, is considered that it is difficult to find out precise solution because of discrete and non-contiguous data structure; therefore, we have decided to find solution of interactive problems by introducing the method of scaling up [13–15], which needs to be revised in the field of education. As this scaling up method should not change the current education system at their university, we have asked instructors and students to participate in experimental practical nursing class and agree to investigate their problems and solutions continuously [16].

2.2 Measuring system

Before starting those practical experiments, we had been developing the measuring system for individual traits [12], regarding human information processing. This system is simulated interactive communication between an instructor (A) and a learner (B) with using ICT (a) → (b) → (c) → (d) (**Figure 4**). In the field of educational technology studies, they call this interaction as learning process. When the learner responses to the instructor (A) after the information or instruction for assignments from the instructor (A) conveyed to her or him, the one session of activity has been considered as coming into effect of learning (**Figure 5**).

From this theory of learning processing, we predicted that language information processing might be the same as each other (**Figure 5**, ①). Then, instead of the instruction or assignment, we decided to use questionnaires of YGPI (Yatabe-Guilford Personality Inventory), which is consisted of 120 short sentences and 12 factors (10 of 120 each), and more, they are composed of two main factors, emotional and non-emotional factors. Subjects are required to choose responses to questionnaires among "yes," "no," or "either," comparing with their daily activities or behavior. The system also measures their response time from the start of presenting the questionnaire to subjects' replies (**Figure 5**, ② and ③). Card has

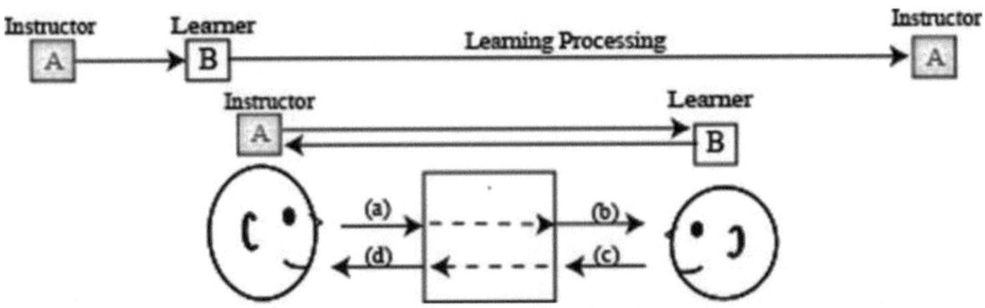

Figure 4.
Learning processing.

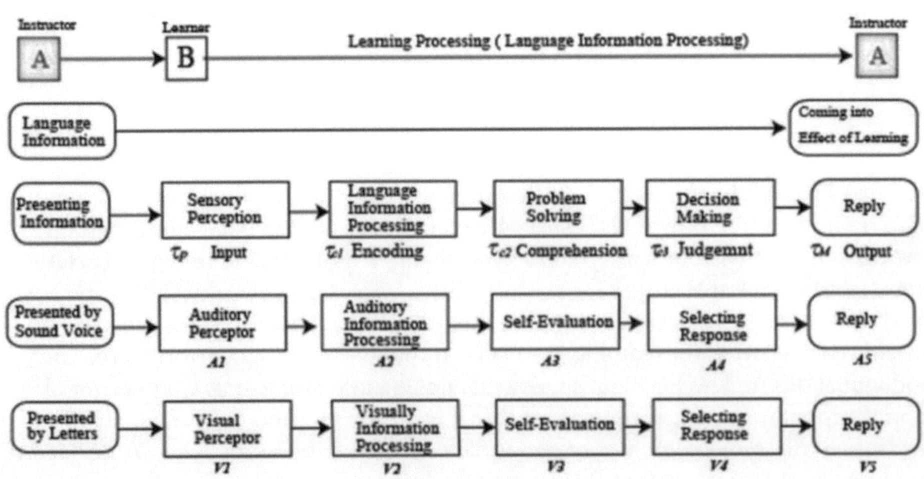

Figure 5.
Human information processing.

introduced the theory that the perceptional system (τ_p), cognitive system (τ_c), and motor system (τ_M) are involved in simple reaction time [17, 18].

Learning Processing = Sensory Perception ⟶ Reply (Coming into Effect of Learning)

ResonseTime $= (\tau_P) + \tau_{c1} + \tau_{c2} + \tau_{c3} + (\tau_M)$ ……… ①

Response Time $= (A1) + A2 + A3 + A4 + (A5)$ ……… ②
(by Sound Voice)

Response Time $= (V1) + V2 + V3 + V4 + (V5)$ ……… ③
(by Letters)

2.3 Hypothesis

As questionnaires would be the same between those presented by sound voice and letters, differences of their response time should be the same, except the duration of comprehension for problem solving (τ_{c2}) and decision making of intention (τ_{c3}), which are considered working as high-order functions. Hence, response time, which is measured in this study, is not the same as simple reaction time but same as complex reaction time. According to the theory of information processing by Card [17, 18], reaction time for encoding by perceptive organs (τ_{c1}) is correlated with the number of words, because of cycling for processing with each elements of the word.

The results of our exploratory experiments (over 100 subjects aged from 13 to 64) have been shown, however, that the system of encoding might not be the same among subjects. Especially, encoding system [19] for letters might be different individually, and the results of preliminary experiments which have been conducted in the same conditions (age, sex, history of education, and environment of experiments) have imprecated the individual differentiation of cognitive system, included encoding.

From these perspectives, we had introduced the model of human information processing (**Figure 5**) into our research. Specifically, it was predicted that there might be individual differences of information processing, depending on contents of questionnaires, between emotional and non-emotional factors [4] because of the encoding system or image schema system (**Figure 5**; A2, V2) [20], which is concerning with conceptualization. Those might have effects on their comprehension (**Figure 5**; A3, V3) or decision making (**Figure 5**; A4, V4) strongly.

Consequently, the model of information processing had been reviled to **Figure 6** which shows two types of cycle: (4) and (5). Along with previous examinations, the criteria would be decided for discriminating each other by analyzing correlation coefficient between response time and duration of reading (listening) or the

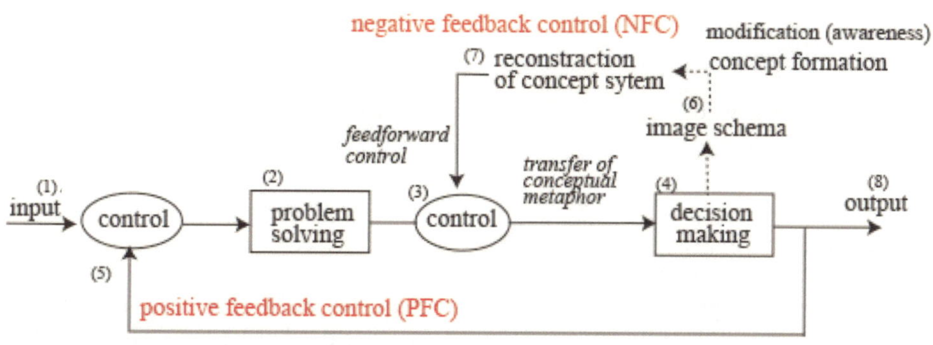

Figure 6.
Model of language information processing system.

number of words, depending on contents; emotional and non-emotional factors. In this chapter, we will examine hypotheses of "dual loop theory" as below.

There might have existed two loops for human information processing: one might be a positive feedback control (PFC) and the other might be a negative feedback control (NFC). Depending on students, which they might choose one during the problem solving would be different and it might be clarified by analyzing the response time, regarding the context of questionnaires.

a. In the case of PFC, Loop of (1)(2)(4)(5), (**Figure 6**), encoded words into symbols might be feedback directly to perceptive organs in order to comprehend the next word along with the context of given each questionnaire. Therefore, this type might have a tendency toward eidetic with short-term memory (STM) to make their decisions in a short time without phonologically silent reading.

b. In the case of NFC, Loop of (1)(2)(4)(6)(7)(3)(4)(8), (**Figure 6**), encoded words into symbols might be feedback control after phonologization with image schema and matching meanings of the words with sound voice by long-term memory (LTM). If there are conflicts between them, s/he might need to modify either one of them; then, the results would be conveyed to the cycle of feedforward control (**Figure 6**; (3)). In this case, they need time to make decision.

c. Most of the students might use both loops to solve problems and make decisions for replies. How they might choose one, depending on questionnaires, would be effects on their performances.

And more over, this tendency might have effects on their personality.

2.4 Methods of experiment

2.4.1 Prototype experiment

2.4.1.1 Purpose

The purpose of prototype experiments is to calibrate the measurement system.

2.4.1.2 Participant

Twenty-eight university students participated in this experiment.

2.4.1.3 Duration

The experiment took place from January to March in 2015.

2.4.1.4 Procedure

The participants were divided into two groups for a counterbalance depending on orders of the way of presentation by sound voice or letters. Prototype experiments are implemented twice to the same participants in the same way and conditions in January and March, for example, the arrangement of laptop displays on the desks and seats in the same room.

2.4.1.5 Data gathering

Each comparative experiment plans to obtain 240 responses and response time per person. Total amount of data should be 6720 for each element.

2.4.2 Practical experiment

2.4.2.1 Purposes

Under the condition of optimized combinations of team members at this time by considering inter personality which is predicted by the result of YGPI and instructors' experiences, the aim is to find out problems remaining in collaborative learning class in order to improve students' performance from another factor.

2.4.2.2 Participants

Ninety-eight new students at university participated in this experiment.

2.4.2.3 Duration

The experiment took place from April in 2015 to March in 2016.

2.4.2.4 Procedure

Beforehand, the instructors had been introduced how to optimize combination of team members in teacher training by using personality types and their experiences. At first, students were explained about the practical experiment and collaborative learning. After obtaining their agreements, they had participated in activities of this experiment, for instance, taking personality testing before starting class, answering questionnaires, collaborative learning in practical nursing class with optimized team members, and so on. Students were required to wear the saddlecloth so that observers and instructors can survey their behavior individually in class.

2.4.2.5 Data gathering

1. The results of performance in class; both low and high stakes assignment;

2. YGPI (response, response time, and evaluation (profile));

3. questionnaires and interviews to instructors and students;

4. interaction among students while they are using LMS (learning management system);

5. record of video in class; and

6. participatory fieldwork.

2.5 Methods of analysis

2.5.1 Quantitative analyses

2.5.1.1 Calibration

The calibration is done by comparing the average of response time to questionnaires by presenting sound voice or letters obtained in prototype experiments in the first and the second time, divided by the number of words.

2.5.1.2 Traits of information processing I

The calibration is done by comparing the average of response time to questionnaires by presenting sound voice or letters obtained in practical experiments in Visual and Auditory types (**Table 1**), divided by the number of words.

2.5.1.3 Traits of information processing II

The calibration is done by comparing scatter diagrams of response time to questionnaires by presenting letters and standard reading time (sound voice) obtained in practical experiments in Eidetic and Adjusting types (**Table 2**), dividing into emotional and non-emotion context (**Table 3**).

2.5.1.4 Evaluation of performance in team

After processing parallel distributions of individual records of performance, low and high stakes assessments, and traits of information processing (**Tables 1** and **2**), a table will be made in order to analyze and evaluate by comparing performances of teams between success and ill-successes team (Team B and Team C).

Traits of Information Processing I	
Visual Type	r <0.3
Auditory Type	r >0.5
Intermidiate Type	0.3=<r <=0.5

Table 1.
Criteria type I.

Traits of Information Processing II	
Eidetic Type	$X = <\mu-\sigma$
Adjusting Type	$X = >\mu+\sigma$
Intermidiate Type	$\mu-\sigma < X < \mu+\sigma$

Table 2.
Criteria type II.

Element of Material	Context	Items	Minimum	Maximm	$\overline{X}$	*SD*
the Number of Characters	Emotional	60	4	20	14.3	4.2
	Non-Emotional	*60*	*4*	*20*	*14.2*	*4.2*
the Length of Time for Reading Item	Emotional	60	0.76	3.2	2.0	0.6
	Non-Emotional	*60*	*0.73*	*3.0*	*2.0*	*0.6*

Table 3.
Comparison of elements between emotion and non-emotion.

2.5.2 Qualitative analyses

After processing parallel distributions of individual traits of information processing (**Tables 1** and **2**), descriptions of answering questionnaires about psychological testing will be compared between two types of presentation and interpersonal communication in class or practical training (Team B and Team C).

Then, their differences will be discussed in order to clarify the effectiveness of collaborative learning.

3. Results

3.1 Prototype experiment

Twenty-eight participants were the same members as the first and the second implementation on the same seat and the same display for each person. The experiments were conducted by representing counter-balanced by order. The results were obtained by analyzing the average of reaction time divided by number of words in a short sentence (**Figure 7**); both sound voice and letters were not significantly different between the first and the second experiments. The total average (first, second) of sound voice was (=2.69, =2.58) and letters (=2.32, =2.20). The correlation coefficients between response time and the number of words were not significantly different between the first and the second experiments, both representing questionnaires by sound voice and letters (**Table 4**).

From these results, it has been proved with reliability that the level of calibration was high enough to reproduce scientifically, regarding our measuring system. Concerning standard deviation, however, letters (*SD* = 0.93, *SD* = 0.85) was larger than sound voice (*SD* = 0.64, *SD* = 0.64) (**Figure 5**). Specifically, when the number of words was higher, the standard deviation of reaction time to letters became

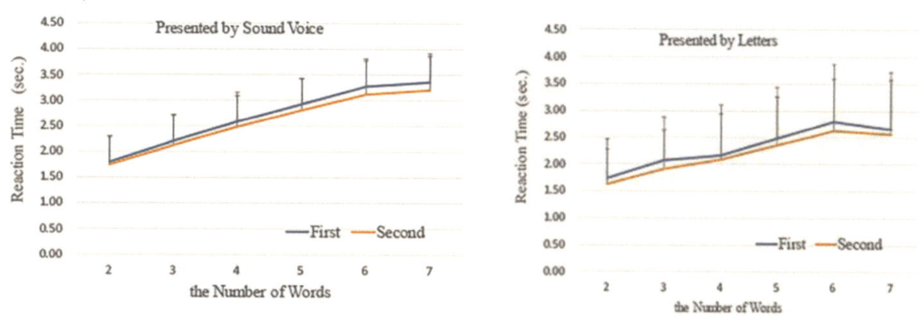

Figure 7.
Comparison of response time between the first and the second experiments (left: presented by sound voice; right: presented by letters).

	Correlation Coefficient					
	Materials of Media					
	Sound Voice			Letters		
	df.	*r*	*t-ratio*	*df.*	*r*	*t-ratio*
First (N=28)	3360	0.70	*n.s.*	3360	0.37	*n.s.*
Second (N=28)	3360	0.68		3360	0.38	

Table 4.
Examination of comparison between the first and the second response time.

larger. This means that there might be individual differences of information processing among students.

3.2 Practical experiment

3.2.1 Quantitative analyses

3.2.1.1 Comparison of traits for information processing I

As we have mentioned in Section 3.1, from the results of prototype experiments, we have proved the reliability and the reproducibility of our measurement system. Then, in a practical experiment, we have used them and gathered data, with the similar way of procedures and conditions applied in the prototype experiments. As the standard deviation of response time presented by letters was larger than those of sound voice, we have checked individual differences of the correlation coefficients between response time and the number of words. Along with the categorization of those correlation coefficients, we have divided students' types as traits of information processing I, Visual type and Auditory type. And then, comparing the average of reaction time between Visual and Auditory type (**Figure 8**), in the case of letters, Visual type (=2.01, SD = 0.92, N = 13) responded significantly faster than Auditory type (=2.65, SD = 0.98, (N = 31)) (**Table 5**) ($t = -21.05$, $r < 0.001$).

3.2.1.2 Comparison of traits for information processing II

Figure 9 shows the different patterns of distributed response time (intermediate type of information processing I) between eidetic (N = 8 of 11) and adjusting type

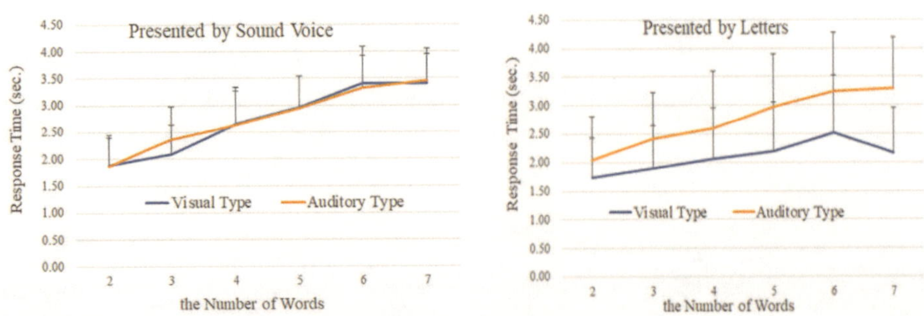

Figure 8.
Comparison of reaction time between Visual and Auditory types (left: presented by sound voice; right presented by letters).

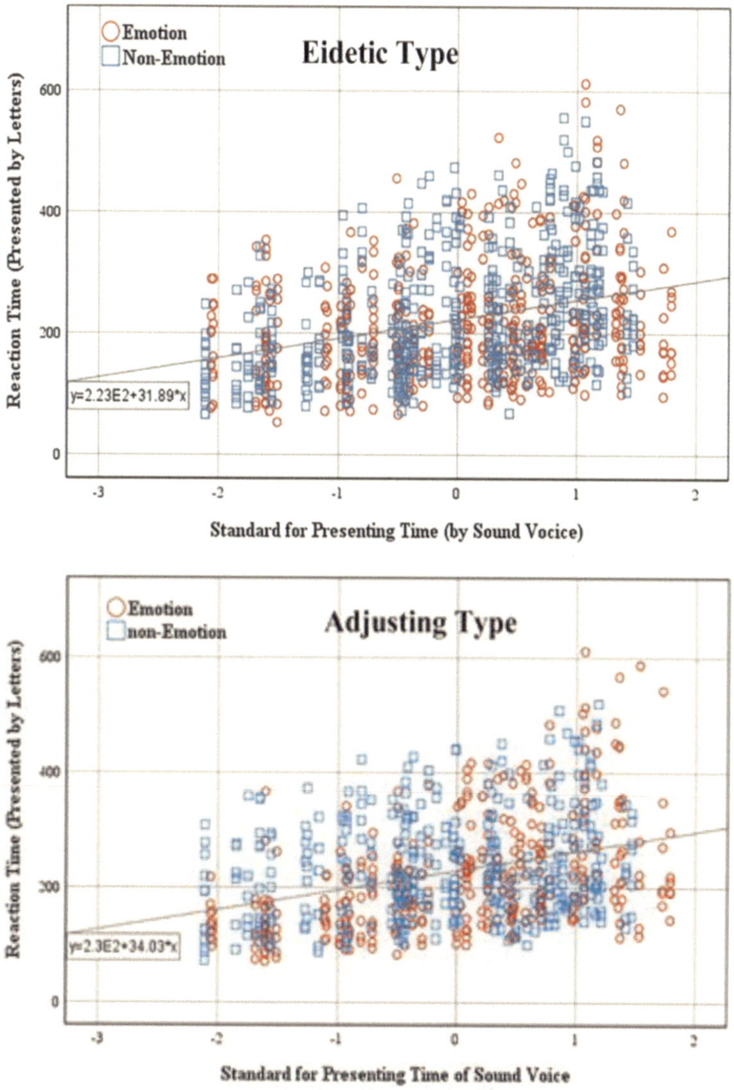

Figure 9.
Comparison of reaction time between emotion and non-emotion (upper: Eidetic type; lower: Adjusting type).

	Comparison of ReactionTime							
	Materials of Media							
Traits of Information Processin I	Sound Voice				Letters			
	$\overline{X}$ *(SD)*	*df.*	*t-ratio*	*t - test*	$\overline{X}$ *(SD)*	*df.*	*t-ratio*	*t - test*
Auditory Type (N=31)	2.64 *(0.89)*	5156	2.12	*	2.65 *(0.98)*	5154	-21.05	***
Visual Type (N=13)	2.70 *(0.82)*				2.01 *(0.92)*			

Table 5.
Results of tests, the significant differences of reaction time between visual and auditory types.

(N = 6 of 10), which were categorized traits by the differences of correlation coefficients between emotional and non-emotional contexts (eidetic type; $X \leq \mu\text{-}\sigma$, Adjusting type; $X \geq \mu + \sigma$) (**Table 2**). In the case of Adjusting type (N = 10), the average of response time of emotional contexts was significantly faster than those of

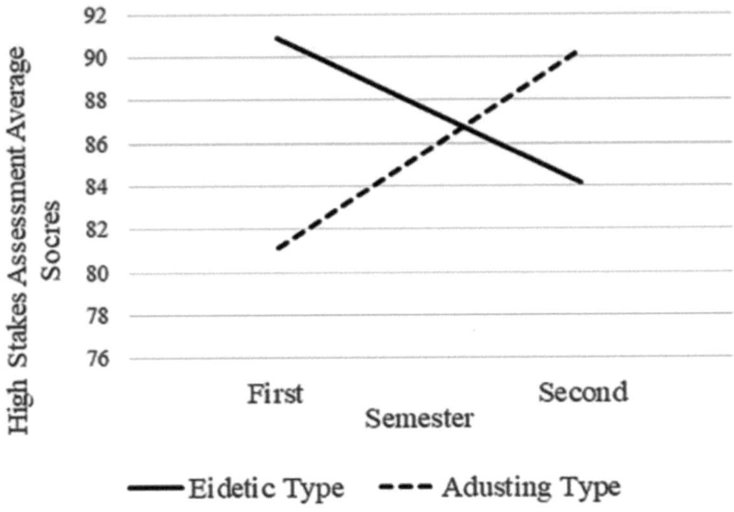

Figure 10.
Comparison of scores first and second semester.

non-emotional contexts. This tendency is found in the patterns of the scatter diagram, which shows distributions of each response time how they diff between emotional and non-emotional contexts. On the other hand, in the case of Eidetic type ($N = 11$), there are no differences between them.

Figure 10 shows the quantitative interaction between two types of students, comparing their scores between the first and the second semesters ($F = 5.3, p < 0.01$). The average of Eidetic type in the first semester was better than that of Adjusting type; however, in the second semester, it was reversed.

3.2.1.3 Comparison of team performance

This phenomenon should be examined in detail, checking whether the statistical results are right or not by seeing individual performances practically. Therefore, we have chosen team members whose team was success or ill-success in low- and high-stakes' assessments. In the case of low-stakes assessments, Team B members' records were shown the best improvement among teams, comparing pre-post test scores. On the other hand, in the case of Team C, their records were the worst in class. Those tests conducted in the first semester, and the average of Team C (=77.5) was lower than Team B (=87.3). In the second semester, traits of the whole tendency of teams were the same; however, looking into individual performances, their tendencies were also the same as **Figure 10**. For instance, both scores of eidetic type; SubB-2 and SubC-2 in the second semester were lower than in the first semester, on the other hand, in the case of Adjusting type, SubB-1 and SubC-3, their scores in the second semester, became much better than those of the first semester.

3.2.2 Qualitative analyses

3.2.2.1 Description

In order to check them from another viewpoint practically, their descriptions of answering questionnaires were compared among types of information processing (Appendix 1 and 2).

Appendix 1 shows descriptive answers to the questionnaire about the comparison between auditory and visual presentation of testing. Two of four students, who are visual type, said that it was easier for them to decide responses or image by sound voice than by letters. On the other hand, all three students of Adjusting type have described their responses through self-evaluation by testing.

In Appendix 2, regarding interpersonal communication, which students are required to obtain in practical field for nursing, all three Adjusting type students have described that they think it is important. The others have described about the interactive communication a little more subjectively.

3.2.2.2 Interview

All four members of Team B were interviewed on September 9th in 2018. SubB-2, however, did not appear at the appointment time. After getting appointment again, she appeared for the interview. She said that similar cases have repeatedly happened because it was nothing unusual to make misread message (which caused missing appointment). Concerning interpersonal communication, it has been difficult for her in collaborative working in the practical field and it was the best condition in 2015 with Team B members.

In the case of SubB-1 and SubB-4, they both have talked about their strategies to communicate interactively in collaborative working, even at the specialized treatment department. It seemed that they were able to cope with any persons and cases.

4. Discussion

4.1 Meaning of clarifying human information processing

There are a significant number of studies, which have been conducted about human information processing in the world [17, 18]. Every study is very important for us; on the other hand, most of them are still vague and unclear, because we need to observe real time while it is working, from outside. It should be difficult, however, to see inside of our mind directly. Therefore, we have developed the measurement of individual traits from cognitive aspects so that we can clarify human information processing and predict their behaviors. I would like to make it a meaningful measurement; however, it is still exploratory research and data analysis.

Although there might be a lot of methods to find out the mechanism of human information processing [21, 22], there should be different approaches from each other to achieve a goal, depending on their own purposes. The end of this study is to improve personalized education, however, both the environments in society and educational field have been changing, which must be a lot of elements and always impact on our cognitive system, in other words, on the way of human information processing. This means that we always need to find out the problems which might be courses of ill-success in education.

For instance, in our study case, we have supported collaborative learning in nursing class, which has been introduced for cutting age electronic equipment. It must help students when they start to work at hospital, coping with electronic equipment. On the other hand, they are required to obtain the skill of interactive communication with patients and coworkers. For this reason, the instructors have introduced the method of collaborative learning, which needs to divide students into teams with four members in each. It seems cumbersome to decide the members of teams, if instructors seek for effective learning, because they would be required to predict students' behaviors by analyzing their data, for instance, individual traits and their needs. Hence, we have begun to support optimizing combination; however, there is no exact solution for it [23]. For those reasons, we have developed the support system or personalized education and learning. This has the measuring system to provide students' data to instructors before starting classes.

As I have mentioned above, however, it has been becoming complicated to combine members of teams. Therefore, if AI doctor or machine would solve this problem by optimizing combination, personalized education and learning would be improved. To achieve this meaningful goal, we need to clarify information processing for interactive communication. This must have synergic effect on AI doctor, care assisting robots and so on, because they need to obtain the ability of interactive communication with people by machine learning.

From these viewpoints, this study and the measuring system for clarifying human information processing must be meaningful to achieve our goal.

4.2 Examination of dual loop theory

We have planned to examine dual loop theory, which I have proposed as hypotheses and implemented experiments, gathered data, and analyzed them. Those ideas were hinted by Card's Model Processor [18], which is a "cognitive model of the user to be employed by the designer in thinking about the human interaction with computer at the interface" and "the Recognize-Act Cycle of the Cognitive Processor," from the view of LTM and STM as a simple reaction time. Although they have introduced this model, they have tried to propose another one (GOES: Goals, Operations, Methods, and Selections) for tasks which can be taken from the half-second level to the two-second level. Approximately, dual loop theory model (**Figure 6**) might be a combination of those two models and we can predict subjects' behavior. Many of such models have been introduced; however, there might be a few to find out individual differences in human information processing.

The idea of this dual loop theory might be similar to the others, however, we seek for finding out individual differences which patters would indicate some types of trait concerning with cognitive behavior.

Although having said that, when the model is examined, we need to use previous studies as references. For instance, by comparing processing between sound voice and letters [24] and cycle reaction time which is proposed by Card [18], we have examined calibration of measuring instrument. From the results of analysis for response time by presenting sound voice have been shown the high level of the calibration from the viewpoints of reliability and the reproducibility (**Figure 7**, left), considering the high correlation coefficient with the number of words which means cycle of response time. On the other hand, in the letter presentation case, it was recognized reproducibility; however, its correlation coefficient with the number of words was not shown high.

From this result, it was predicted that individual differences clearly among students concerning the way of silent reading. Then, categorized types of trait (visual or auditory type) by strengthening of the correlation coefficient between response time and the number of words or duration of reading aloud. There are no differences between the two types of reaction time represented questionnaires by sound voice, but recognized significantly differences by letters (**Figure 8** under **Table 5**). Students of Auditory type have needed time longer than those of Visual type from starting to silent reading to making decision (**Figure 5**). This means that the auditory type might tend to process a word and a sentence with phonologization, using LTM or NFC loop; conversely, the visual type tends to process directly encoding symbol using STM or PFC loop.

From these results of analyses, the hypotheses [a] and [b] have been proved, and next hypothesis [c] should be examined. It was predicted that depending on the context of sentences, we might process them with different ways, PFC or NFC Loop. One hundred twenty psychological questionnaires were used as a task for one session, but they consisted of mainly two types of contexts, emotion and non-emotion. From the previous studies, when the emotional context is processed, it is considered that we tend to use STM because the effect of emotion on hippocampal-dependent memory consolidation [25, 26]. Then, the categorization of types concerning contexts is performed, Eidetic [27] and Adjusting type, depending on the differentiation of correlation coefficients between emotional or non-emotional contexts (**Table 2**). In the case of adjusting type, the differentiation of response time was clear, and the average of response time to emotional contexts is significantly faster than non-emotional ones. This means that students of Adjusting type might change their strategies to read silently and make decision depending on contexts. In the case of emotional contexts, they might use STM or PFC; on the other hand, in non-emotional contexts, their correlation coefficient is higher and much longer time spent from starting silent reading to making decision [28, 29]. This means that they might read silently with phonologization of words, referring concepts of words meaning by sound voice with image schema. This information processing might help them to reflect on their comprehension is right or not, which is considered negative feedback control (NFC).

From these results, we have proved hypothesis (c); however, we would like to examine more details for this hypothesis.

4.3 Relevance between individual differences and personality

Two teams were selected from the aspect of low stakes assessments (highest and lowest teams, assessing for ability of conceptual metaphor and collaboration), in order to examine more in detail from the aspect of individual differences (**Table 7**). It is easy to compare the improvement performances among students' traits and records or between teams by parallel processing and analyses. The result of the comparison of the average scores between Eidetic and Adjusting types and between first and second semesters has been examined this parallel processing and analyses, which have shown matching with each other.

Moreover, the comparison of those examinations between results of scores and descriptions of students (Appendix 1 and 2) by parallel processing has shown their matching. From this viewpoint, whether those results are matching with the evaluation of personality, regarding the factors of lack of objectivity (O Factor) and lack of cooperativeness (Co Factor) among 12 factors (Appendix 3). Students of Adjusting type (SubB-1, SabB-4, and SubC-3) have taken low scores for both factors; in other words, they are evaluated as objectivity and cooperativeness are strong. On the other hand, students of eidetic type (SubB-3 and SubC2) have taken high score in both factors, comparing with the former students, which means they are subjective and a little bit uncooperative.

Consequently, we might be also able to predict their behavior from traits of information processing. Though the results of our experiments have been proven useful, they are complicated for us. In addition to it, instructors must be busy to prepare other instructions for students. From these reasons, AI machine or doctor which might be able to obtain machine learning is expected and prospected for matching members of team by optimizing combinations.

5. Conclusions

In this chapter, dual loop theory, which consisted of two kinds of feedback control, concerning with human information processing, was proposed (**Figure 6**) and examined by analyzing the results of experiments. The data were gathered students' response time, using psychological questionnaires (**Figures 4** and 5) and their records of performances in collaborative learning class and analyzed by the way of parallel distributed processing. The results were as follows:

1. The prototype experiments were conducted by representing counter-balanced by order. The results of analyzing the average of reaction time divided by number of words in a short sentence (**Figure** 7) in both sound voice and letters were not significantly different between the first and the second experiments. Therefore, it has been proved with reliability that the level of calibration was high enough to reproduce scientifically, regarding our measuring system.

2. The response time to questionnaires of sound voice presentation was strongly correlated to the number of words which consist of a short sentence of questionnaires. In presenting letters case, the average of correlation coefficients was weaker and dispersed than those of sound voice (**Figure** 7). From these results, it was supposed that there were individual differences during information processing while students were reading silently. Then, their response time was categorized by the strength of correlation coefficients with the number of words (**Tables 1** and 2).

It was found out that the average of response time depending on types was different between each other. In the case of Auditory type, the average of response time was significantly longer than those of Visual type (**Table** 5 and **Figure** 8).

3. Next, when the sentences were divided into two categories, emotion and non-emotion, there were found different phenomena among students, regarding

Traits of Information Processing Ⅱ	Reaction Time / *second* (SD)		t-test		
	Lerres		df.	t-ratio	siguificant probability
	Emotional	Nonemotional			
Adjusting Type (N=10)	2.27 *(0.27)*	2.44 *(0.32)*	1198	2.98	0.003 ***
EideticType (N=11)	2.27 *(0.42)*	2.35 *(0.40)*	1317	1.55	0.121

Table 6.
Results of tests, the significant differentiation of reaction time between emotion and non-emotion context for Adjusting type.

				Low Stakes Assessment (Group Work)							High Stakes Assessment		
Team	Pertici-pant	Traits of information processing		pre test			post test			differ-ence	semester		differ-ence
		I	Ⅱ	Q2	Q3	all	Q2	Q3	all		First	Second	
Team B	SubB-1	inter-mediate	Adjusting	2	0	2	5	5	10	8	79	97	18
	SuaB-2	Visual	Eidetic	0	0	0	5	5	10	10	93	91	-2
	SubB-3	Visual	inter-mediate	0	0	0	5	5	10	10	86	91	5
	SubB-4	inter-mediate	Adjusting	0	0	0	4	4	8	8	91	97	6
Team C	SubC-1	Visual	inter-mediate	5	5	10	5	0	5	-5	65	78	13
	SubC-2	inter-mediate	Eidetic	5	4	9	5	0	5	-4	86	78	-8
	SubC-3	inter-mediate	Adjusting	3	3	6	5	0	5	-1	71	92	21
	SubC-4	Visual	inter-mediate	2	2	4	4	3	7	3	88	92	4

Table 7.
Comparison scores between teams.

traits of information processing type (**Figure 9**). In the case of Adjusting type, the average of response time for emotional contexts was significantly faster than that of non-emotional contexts (**Table 6**).

4. Therefore, the average scores of students' records were compared between Eidetic and Adjusting types. The result has shown the quantitative interaction between them (**Figure 10**).

5. Moreover, we have examined whether those individual differences are connected to other students' performances (**Table** 7, Appendix 1 and 2), and then, checking the verification of the criteria which classified traits both of personality and cognitive features (Appendix 3).

6. Finally, we have discussed on hypotheses (2.3), from three aspects: meaning of clarifying human information processing, the examination of dual loop theory, and the relevance between individual differences and personality. In conclusion, the feature of Adjusting type has been shown their way of information processing by both positive and negative feedback controls, comparing the other type of students, depending on the context. In addition to this result, we have checked their performances, descriptions, and interviews practically.

We need to examine this theory furthermore and optimize the combination of members in order to communicate interactively among students and instructors. Eventually, those results would help the modern style machine learning of artificial intelligent to predict human behavior depending on types and consequently improve their interactive communication with human beings.

In conclusion, dual loop theory would be expected to help us to understand the system of human information processing and predict our behavior according to its patterns. It would be also applicable widely to the machine learning system, for instance, AI doctor and assistive robots which requires the interactive communication with human.

Acknowledgements

The author is grateful to Dr. Kiyoko Tokunaga and participants for collaboration in our practical research.

Appendix 1

Participant	Traits of Information Processing		Experiments (Comparison of questionnaires between sound voice and letters)
			Are there any changes in your mind?
SubB-1	Mid	Adj	After I had been asked questions which I had never been care about before, I have begun to consider anew about myself.
SuaB-2	Vis	Eid	(no response)
SubB-3	Vis	Mid	I had been able to image easier from questionnaires with representing sound voice than letters, because I had to rearrange them for comprehension in the case of silent reading.
SubB-4	Mid	Adj	I had begun to consider afresh about myself what sort of person I am.
SubC-1	Vis	Mid	It was an opportunity for me to think about myself after I had asked about myself both by sound voice and letters questionnaires.
SubC-2	Mid	Eid	After I had expressed me afresh in words, I had recognized by myself what kind person I am.
SubC-3	Mid	Adj	I thought I need to consider about myself anew.
SubC-4	Vis	Mid	There were nothing especially. I had response to questionnaires easier by sound voice than letters.

Appendix 2

Participant	Traits of Information Processing		Interpersonal Communication Are there anything to become aware in practical class or training?
SubB-1	Mid	Adj	It is very important to communicate with patients for care, because it might make an impact on them psychologically and physically.
SuaB-2	Vis	Eid	(no response)
SubB-3	Vis	Mid	There were increased opportunities to compare both good and bad points between me and people sounding me through group working and sessions, and then I have a feeling of myself. And then, I thought I would like to increase my confidence a little bit more.
SubB-4	Mid	Adj	I have recognized again that it is important to communicate with patients in any cases when we would like to convey our ideas in conversation because I think it is easy to change impression depending on our expressions or manners of speaking.
SubC-1	Vis	Mid	After I had aware of nurses, I thought that communication is important.
SubC-2	Mid	Eid	Nurses had changed the manner of speaking depending on patients.
SubC-3	Mid	Adj	I had found that it is important to exchange information with each other so that we are able to perform better practice in class or training.
SubC-4	Vis	Mid	It was more difficult to communicate with patients than I had thought, especially with difficulty to speak. I had aware that we are able to communicate with each other not only by words but also facial expression.

Appendix 3

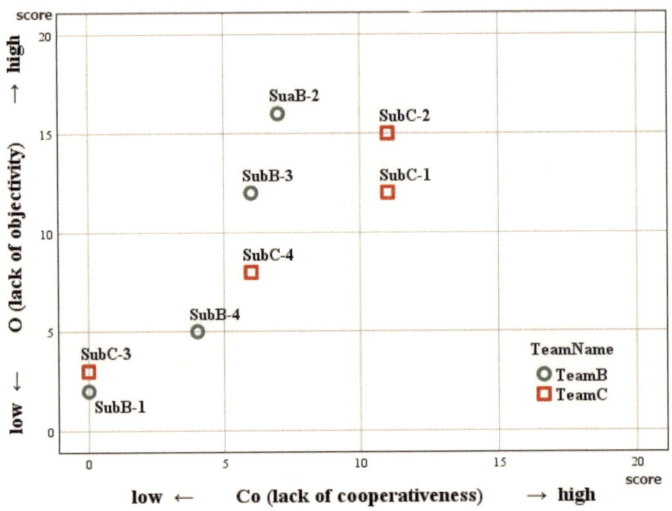

Author details

Keiko Tsujioka
Institute for Psychological Testing, Osaka, Japan

*Address all correspondence to: keiko_tsujioka@sinri.co.jp

References

[1] Tsujioka K. Development of support system modeled on robot suit HAL for personalized education and learning. EITT, Society of International Chinese and Education Technology, IEEE. 2017: 337-338

[2] Tsujioka B, Sonohara T, Yatabe T. A factorial study of the temperament of Japanese College male students by the Yatabe-Guilford personality. Psychologia. 1957;**3**:110-119

[3] Bulck S, Alea N. A tale of three functions: The self-reported autobiographical memory. Social Cognition. 2005;**23**(1):91-117

[4] Tsujioka K. A Study of the Impact of Audio or Visual Media on Decisions in Japanese: Comparing response and reaction times in tasks between emotionality and introversion-extroversion. Annuals of Educational Studies, Osaka University. 2011;**16**:33-44

[5] Tsujioka K. Toward clarifying human information processing: A case study of big data analysis in education. In: Karwowski W, Ahram T, editors. IHSI 2019, AISC 903. Springer Nature. 2019. pp. 1-6. DOI: 10.1007/978-3-030-11051-2_58

[6] Tsujioka K. Toward Clarifying Human Information Processing by Analyzing Big Data: Making Criteria for Individual Traits in Digital Society. [Online First] IntechOpen; DOI: 10.5772/intechopen.86037

[7] Tsujioka KA. Case study of using ICT in education with big data analysis of learners' traits: Toward clear human information processing. Human Interface. 2018:589-594

[8] Kawato M. Internal models for motor control and trajectory planning. Current Opinion in Neurobiology. 1999;**9**:718-727

[9] Kawato M, Furuwaka K, Suzuki R. A hierarchical neural network model for the control and learning of voluntary movements. Biological Cybernetics. 1987;**56**:1-17

[10] Tsujioka K. A Case Study of ICT Used by Big Data Processing in Education: Discuss on Visualization of RE Research Paper, ICIET. Association for Computing Machinery; 2018. ISBN: 978-1-4503-4791

[11] Tsujioka, K. A Case Study of Using Big Data Processing in Education: The Method of Matching Members by Optimizing Collaborative Learning Environment. [Online First] IntechOpen; 2019. DOI: 10.5772/intechopen.85526

[12] Guetzkow H, Gyr J. An analysis of conflict in decision making groups. Human Relations. 1954;**7**:367-381

[13] Dede C. Scaling up: Evolving innovations beyond ideal settings to challenging contexts of practice. In: Sawyer RK, editor. The Cambridge Handbook of the Learning Sciences. Cambridge University Press; 2006. pp. 551-565

[14] Clarke J, Dede C. Design for scalability: A case study of the River City curriculum. Journal of Science Education and Technology. 2009;**18**: 353-365. DOI: 10.1007/s10956-009-9156-4

[15] Clarke J, Dede C, Ketelhut DJ, Nelson B, Bowman C. A design-based research strategy to promote scalability for educational innovations. Educational Technology. 2006;**46**(3):27-36

[16] Nelson BC, Ketelhut DJ, Clark J, Dieterle E, Dede C, Elandson B. Robust design strategies for scaling educational innovations; the River City case study.

In: Shelton BE, Wiley D, editors. The Educational Design and Use of Computer Simulation Games. Rotterdam: The Netherlands Sense Press; 2007. pp. 224-246

[17] Card SK. The Psychology of Human-Computer Interaction. Lawrence Erlbaum Associates, Inc; 2008. ISBN 0-89859-243-7

[18] Newell A, Card SK. The prospects for psychological science in human-computer interaction. In: Human Computer-Interaction. Vol. 1. Lawrence Erlbaum Associates Inc; 1985. pp. 209-242

[19] Baldwin MW. Relational schemas and the processing of social information. Psychological Bulletin. 1992;**112**(3): 461-484

[20] Buchanan TW, Lutz K, Mirzade S, Specht K, Shah NJ, Zilles J, et al. Recognition of emotional prosody and verbal components of spoken language: An fMRI study. Cognitive Brain Research. 2000;**9**:227-238

[21] Baddeley A, Thomson N, Buchman M. Word length and structure of short-term memory. Journal of Verbal Language and Verbal Behavior. 1959;**14**:575-589

[22] Baker R, Simons G. Educational data minding and learning analytics. In: Sawyer RK, editor. The Cambridge Handbook of the Learning Sciences. 2nd ed. Cambridge University Press; 2014. pp. 253-271

[23] Crescenzi P, Kann V. Approximation on the web: A compendium of NP optimization problems. In: Rolim J, editor. Randomization and Approximation Techniques in Computer Science. RANDOM 1997. Lecture Notes in Computer Science. Vol. 1269. Berlin, Heidelberg: Springer; 1997

[24] Rohde DLT, Plaut DC. Connectionist models of language processing. Cognitive Studies. 2003; **10**(1):10-28. DOI: 10.11225/jcss.10.10

[25] Buchanan TW, Adolphs R. The neuroanatomy of emotional memory in humans. In: Reisberg D, Hertel P, editors. Memory and Emotion. Oxford University Press; 2003

[26] Buchanan TW. Retrieval emotional memories. Psychological Bulletin. 2007; **133**(5):761-779

[27] Allport GL. The eidetic image and the after image. The American Journal of Psychology. 1928;**40**(3):418-425. DOI: 10.2307/1414458. Available at: https://www.jstor.org/stable/1414458

[28] Pisoni DB, Garber EE. Lexical memory in visual and auditory modalities: The case for a common mental lexicon. In: ICSLP-1990. 1990. pp. 401-404

[29] Amano S, Kondo T, Kakehi K. Modality dependency of familiarity ratings of Japanese words. Perception & Psychophysics. 1995;**57**(5):598-603

Section 3

Rehabilitation Systems

Chapter 5

Technical Contributions to the Quality of Telerehabilitation Platforms: Case Study—ePHoRt Project

Patricia Acosta-Vargas, Janio Jadán-Guerrero, Cesar Guevara, Sandra Sanchez-Gordon and Tania Calle-Jimenez

Abstract

This chapter proposes three main technical contributions for the development of a telerehabilitation platform, named ePHoRT, for patients recovering from hip surgery. The first contribution is the application of a diffuse 3D model for the detection of rehabilitation exercises after hip surgery. The model applies fuzzy logic, which allows identifying in real time if a patient is performing a right or wrong movement, assisted by an avatar in 3D. The avatar copies the movements of the patient through a Kinect camera. The second contribution involves the proposal of an iterative method to improve the usability of telerehabilitation platforms along the development life cycle. The proposed method involves the use of an inspection method and includes protocols and instruments. This method has been validated in the ePHoRT project. Finally, the chapter describes accessibility guidelines for educational resources. It proposes accessibility standards for the content of educational resources in video and PDF formats in the telerehabilitation platform according to the Web Content Accessibility Guidelines (WCAG).

Keywords: eHealth, telemedicine, telerehabilitation, hip surgery patients, fuzzy logic, usability, accessibility, educational resources, WCAG

1. Introduction

The ePHoRT platform allows hip replacement patients to perform part of the rehabilitation treatment at home and communicate the evolution of the recovery process to the physiotherapist. The ePHoRT platform has a "practice module" organized into three stages that are meaningful for the patient's recovery process. These stages are characterized by a growing level in the intensity of the exercises. Stage 1 is carried out during the week following the surgery and consists mainly of exercises performed lying down. Foot rehabilitation movements begin in stage 2 (the second week after surgery). Finally, stage 3 is characterized by functional exercises, which consist of preparing the patient to recover a regular walk. The ePHoRT platform is in the design stage and follows a process of agile and collaborative development focused on the user.

2. Application of a diffuse 3D model for the detection of rehabilitation exercises after hip surgery

At the present time, it has been seen that intelligent systems embrace a large number of daily life tasks and activities of the society. The objective of these systems is to solve a variety of existing problems in society more efficiently and with accurate results. One of the characteristics of these systems is the interaction between the user and the computer [1], which allows the optimal handling of these systems intuitively.

The present work proposes the development of a virtual representation of the body structure of a patient who performs rehabilitation exercises. This digital representation is called avatar [2], which duplicates the movement of the human being that has been detected by a Kinect camera from Microsoft's Xbox One.

The captured movements are imitated by the avatar and executed in real time. Subsequently, if the patient performs an incorrect exercise, the system will show an alert with the part of the body where it is moving wrongly, with colors that help the patient's interaction. A detector subsystem applies the diffuse logic technique that identifies the execution of rehabilitation exercises; this allows the avatar to be a means of interaction between human and computer.

In the work presented by Ichim et al. [2], the development of three-dimensional facial avatars is detailed. The system detects facial expression from a template and a sequence of recorded images through an optimization that integrates the tracking of expression characteristics. This study helps the design of new applications of computer animation as well as online communication based on personalized avatars. In addition, demonstrations of several applications in real time that verify the process of avatars creation are presented.

In the work published by Pavone et al. [3], the application of immersive virtual reality and electroencephalography recording is presented to explore the avatar's error incorporation when it is viewed from a one-person perspective. The avatar activates the error monitoring system in a patient's brain and helps its development. The results show that immersive virtual reality can obtain optimal results with the application of an artificial agent. These tools improve the fine-tuning learning (motor skills), up to critical social functions (reading or anticipating the other people's intentions).

The study published by Belal et al. [4] presents the study of pulse oximetry. It is a technology used to monitor oxygen saturation in neonates and pediatric patients. The equipment that measures the pulse oximetry is not precise, whereby they generate false alarms. This study proposes the development of a knowledge-based system that uses fuzzy logic to classify plethysmogram pulses into two categories: valid and artifact. The model correctly classified 82% of the valid segments and 93% of the distorted segments.

The study developed by Guevara et al. [5] proposes a model of real-time movement detection of patients of rehabilitation from hip surgery. The model applies the fuzzy logic technique to identify correct and incorrect movements in the performance of rehabilitation exercises using the motion capture device called Kinect of Xbox One. It proposes an algorithm that works with a multivariable logic model. The diffuse model identifies movements of the patient during the performance of rehabilitation exercises. On the other hand, a 3D avatar is applied, which copies and graphically displays the real-time exercises performed by the patients.

2.1 Data analysis

The information used for the avatar development was obtained from the capture of body points by the Kinect camera of the Xbox One (**Figure 1**). In this study, we gained information of four patients who have gone through hip surgery. This

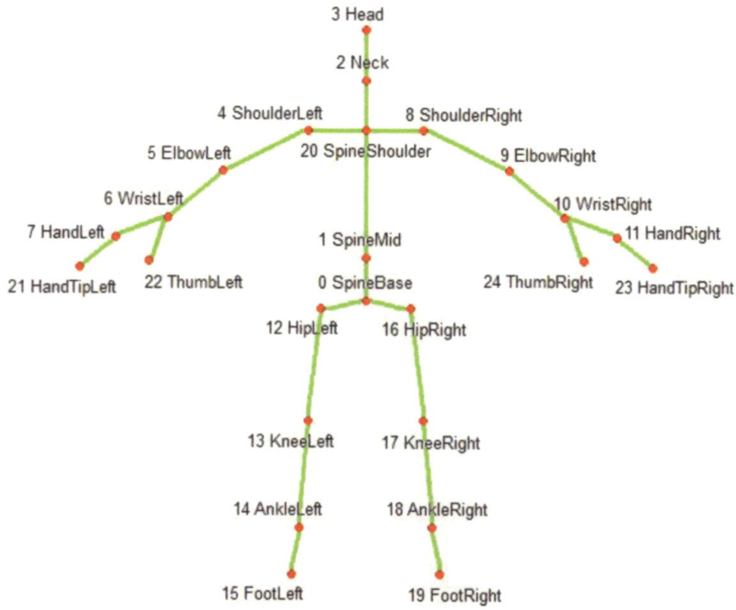

Figure 1.
Body points captured by Microsoft's Kinect [6].

information was collected during 5 weeks of rehabilitation, with high-, medium-, and low-difficulty exercises. Patients performed a set of exercises correctly and incorrectly, which enabled the avatar real movement.

The detected points were 25, the same ones that can identify any movement in three dimensions. For this reason, the database contains 75 attributes. An information preprocessing has been carried out to identify the relevant information, eliminating repeated data as well as noise.

The attribute selection for the algorithm has been identified as 18 essential points of the skeleton detected by the Kinect Xbox One. The specific points are 0y, 6x, 6y, 10x, 10y, 12x, 12y, 13x, 13y, 14x, 14y, 15x, 15y, 16x, 16y, 17x, 17y, and 19x. These points determine the movement in a more detailed way, allowing depth and opening angle detection. The points selected for the front step exercise are those shown in **Figure 2** as well as in the lateral step exercise, as shown in **Figure 3**.

2.2 Proposed model

The proposed model uses the points identified in the previous section. With this information, we will calculate the speed and angle of the limb opening that have performed the rehabilitation exercises correctly. This information is vital to build the diffuse model and to determine the patient's correct posture while performing the exercise (arms, shoulders, and head), as well as the execution speed and the opening angle.

2.3 Limb opening angle calculation

To calculate the angle of the limbs, we identified starting points defined as $B(X_i, Y_i)$ and ending point $C(X_j, Y_j)$. The value of the angle between points B and C is defined as α, as shown in **Figure 4**. In the same way, the execution speed defined as ρ will be calculated.

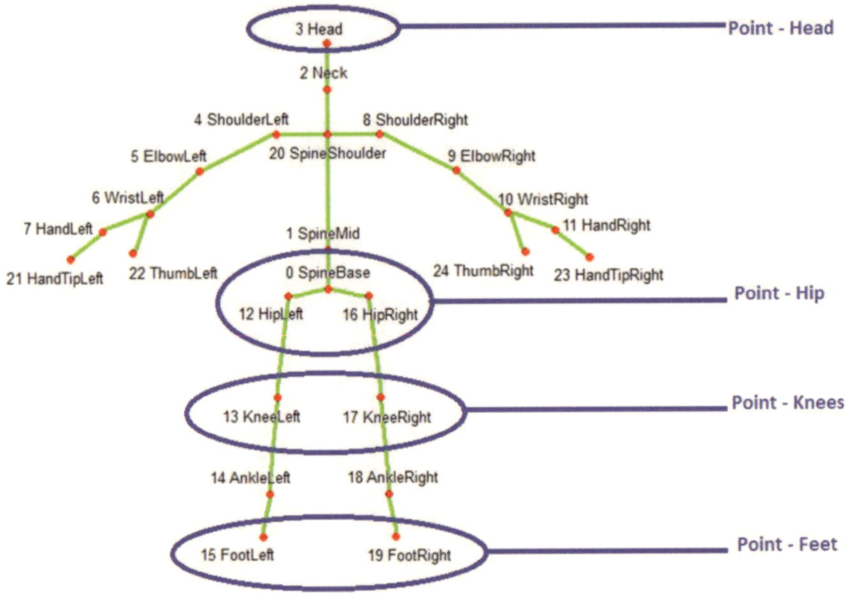

Figure 2.
Selected points for front step exercise.

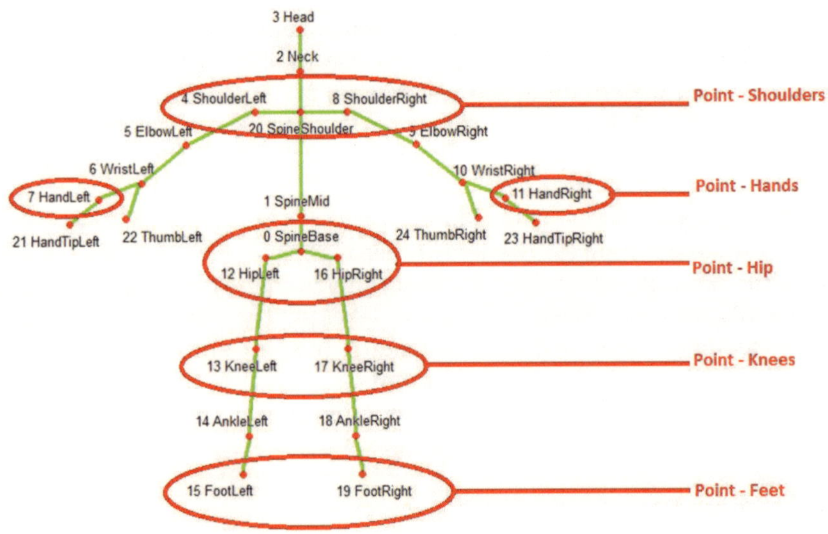

Figure 3.
Selected points for lateral step exercise.

To complete the movement modeling of the limbs, it has been based on **Table 1**, which details when the rehabilitation exercise is performed in a low, correct, or high way.

The diffuse model is based on **Table 1** variables, where the patient's correct movement is obtained while performing each of the rehabilitation exercises. Any exercise that is outside the range identified as "good" will be detected as "poorly executed exercise," where the system will give an alert that the variable is being performed incorrectly. The diffuse model is presented in **Figure 5**.

The following section describes the avatar design and development process in three dimensions using the Blender tool, based on the information captured from

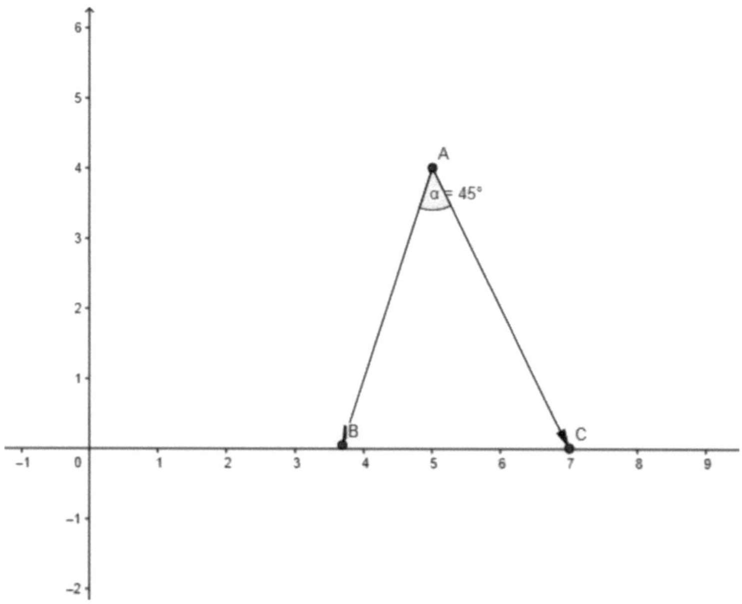

Figure 4.
Limb opening angle calculation.

	Low		Good		High	
	Min	Max	Min	Max	Min	Max
Angle of legs (degrees) α	0	24	25	45	46	90
Hip movement (cm) μ	-	-	0	10	11	20
Shoulder movement (cm) β	-	-	0	10	11	20
Head movements (cm) δ	-	-	0	10	11	20
Execution speed (cm/s) ρ	20	30	10	19	5	9

Table 1.
Rules to determine correct or incorrect movement of rehabilitation exercises.

several patients who performed physiotherapy exercises over a period of 4 weeks. The exercises performed in this data collection phase were lateral step and front step (**Figure 6**).

The following section describes how the patient's avatar was designed. This avatar will imitate the patient's movements during rehabilitation.

2.4 Avatar development

The avatar design is fundamentally based on the skeleton in **Figure 1**, which describes all the points detected by the Kinect. This design was then loaded to Blender and the scale of the header image adjusted, as shown in **Figure 7**.

To generate a three-dimensional avatar was necessary to generate two 3D windows (two windows for the avatar frontal and lateral view), as can be seen in **Figure 8**.

For the avatar design, the work has to be simultaneous with the modeling of two avatars, both doctor (male) and nurse (female). This development has been implemented with all the characteristics of clothing, ethnicity, and age of the employees

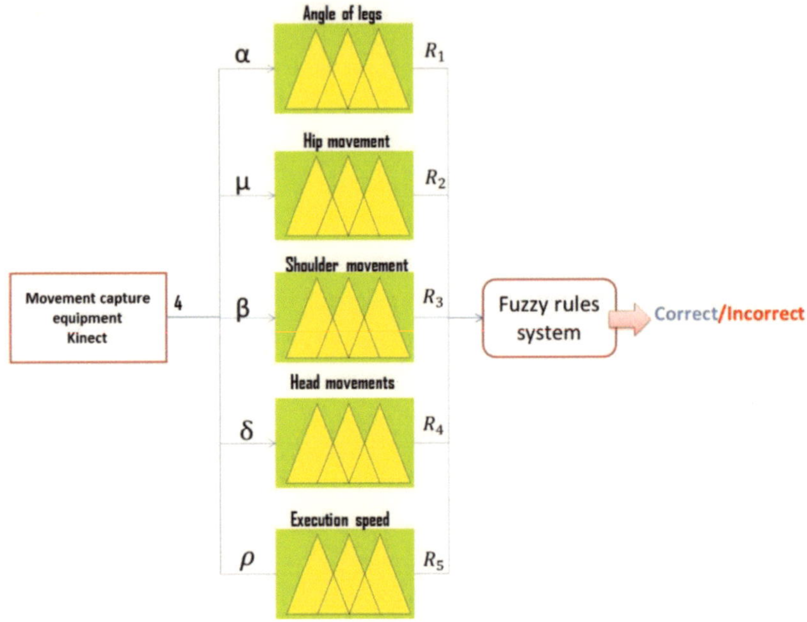

Figure 5.
Diffuse model for exercise detection in telerehabilitation [5].

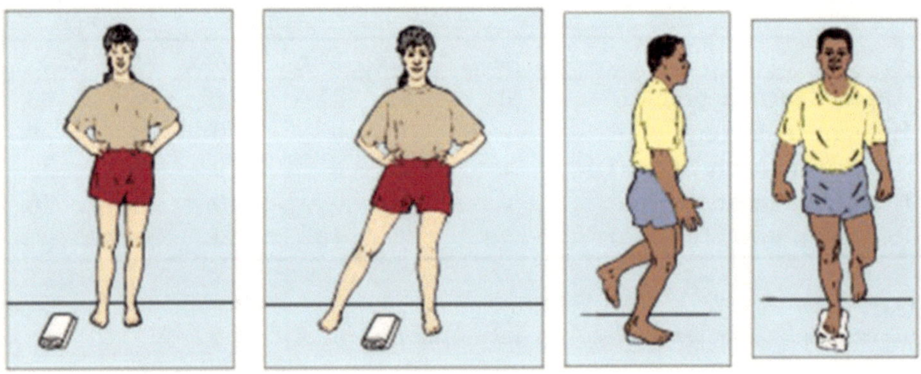

Figure 6.
Exercise images for lateral step and front step.

that work in a health center, as shown in **Figure 9**. Part of the body of the avatar is designed with proportional measures as well as with skin and clothing textures in order to have a real shape and contour avatar.

Finally, we obtained two functional avatars that will imitate the patient's movements in three dimensions. These avatars will be able to move thanks to an interconnected system between the Kinect and a diffuse model of detection of speed, rhythm, and angles of movement of each of the 75 corporal points. This diffuse model is connected to the avatar through Python language and Java for online movement, which results in efficient response time.

2.5 Implementation

The telerehabilitation model implementation was obtained with N-layer development architecture of the intelligent system. As shown in **Figure 10**, the architecture covers layers such as a database, application server, web server, and application.

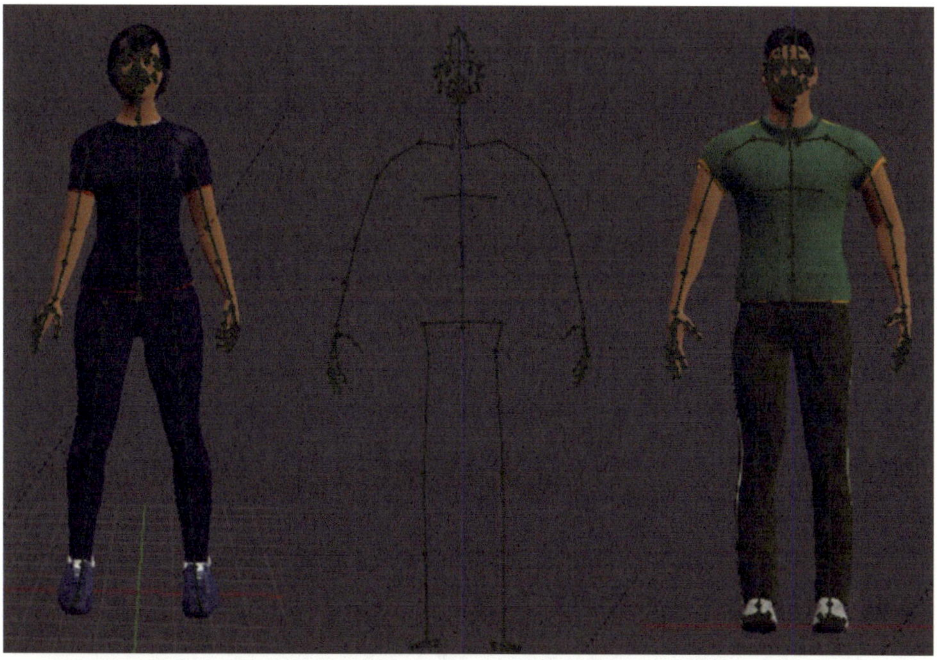

Figure 7.
Skeleton detected by Kinect uploaded to the Blender tool.

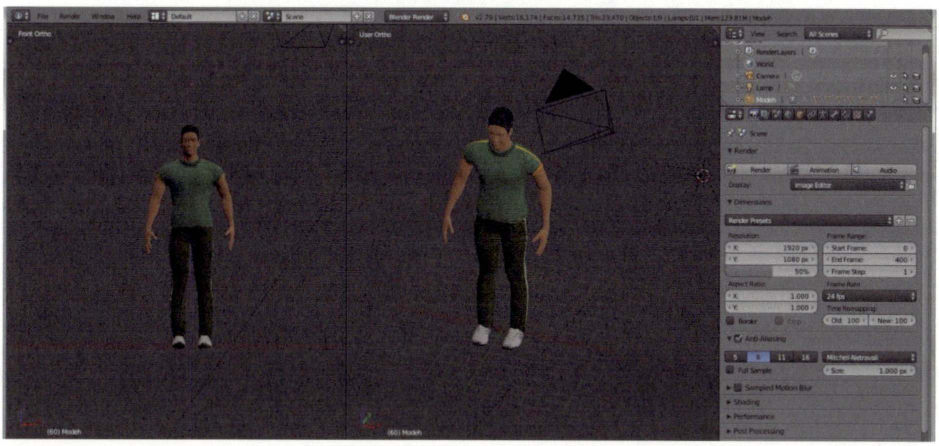

Figure 8.
Front view and side view windows of the doctor avatar.

The database server contains the patient's information (name, age, gender, and medical history). It also contains the data of each of the rehabilitation exercises performed correctly. This allows that during the execution of a movement in the rehabilitation, the system can identify if the patient is doing the exercises correctly or incorrectly. The application server is the one that contains all the programming to register the information in the database, interconnection with devices (Kinect), consumption of complementary applications (avatar in Blender), and system security. The application server's architecture is presented in **Figure 11**. This architecture is service-oriented, due to the fact that many add-ons to the system are not executed in Java.

In the business rules layer is the diffuse model of detection of rehabilitation exercises. The implemented model uses the points captured by the Kinect, to later calculate the angles and maximum and minimum speeds of the limbs, so that the

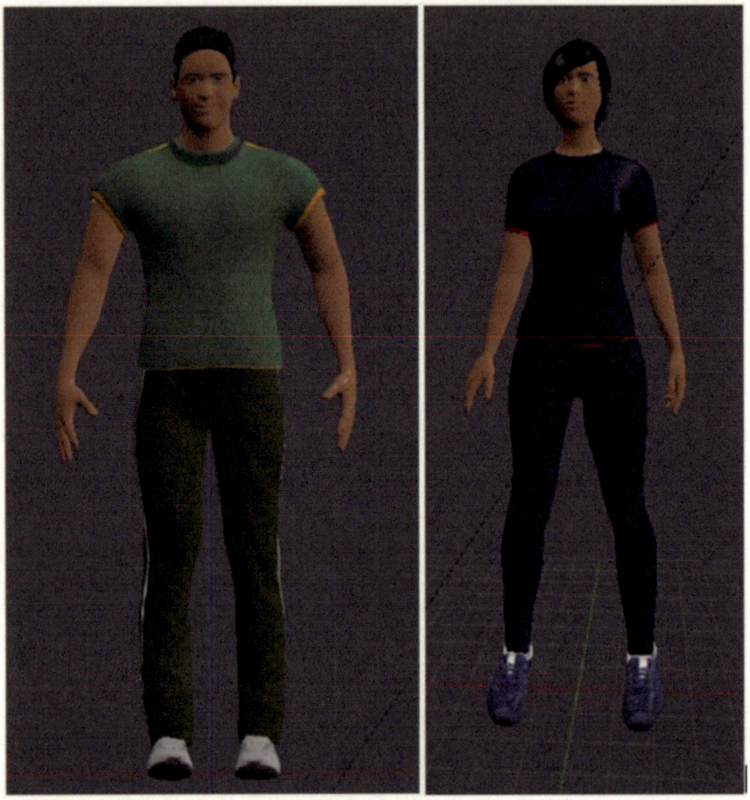

Figure 9.
Doctor avatar (man) and nurse avatar (woman).

patient can perform a correct rehabilitation exercise. In addition, it detects the optimal distances of movement for complementary points such as the arms, shoulders, and head. To calculate the appropriate angles for each of the exercises was necessary to identify the starting point $B(X_i, Y_i)$, the ending point $C(X_j, Y_j)$, and the value of the angle α of the triangle formed by the trajectory.

The diffuse model shown in **Figure 5** detects the opening angle between the legs, hip movement, shoulder movement, head movement, and the speed at which the exercise was executed. With these variables, it can be efficiently determined in real time if an exercise has been performed correctly or incorrectly [7, 8].

While the patient is performing the exercises, the avatar copies and performs the patient's movements in real time, which makes it easier to graphically identify the exact moment of an incorrect movement. The system's graphical interface developed in Java and hosted in an Apache Tomcat web server allows user's access around the world through an Internet domain.

The web application is deployed by the user's device, which must be connected to the Kinect motion capture device, that allows it to be connected to the system and records the patient's movement in real time. The system requires a bandwidth greater than 2 MB/s Internet access so that the application can perform optimal results.

2.6 Results

The results obtained in this proposal have revealed that the exercise detection rate is 97.42% with a false-positive percentage of 2.58%, as shown in **Table 2**.

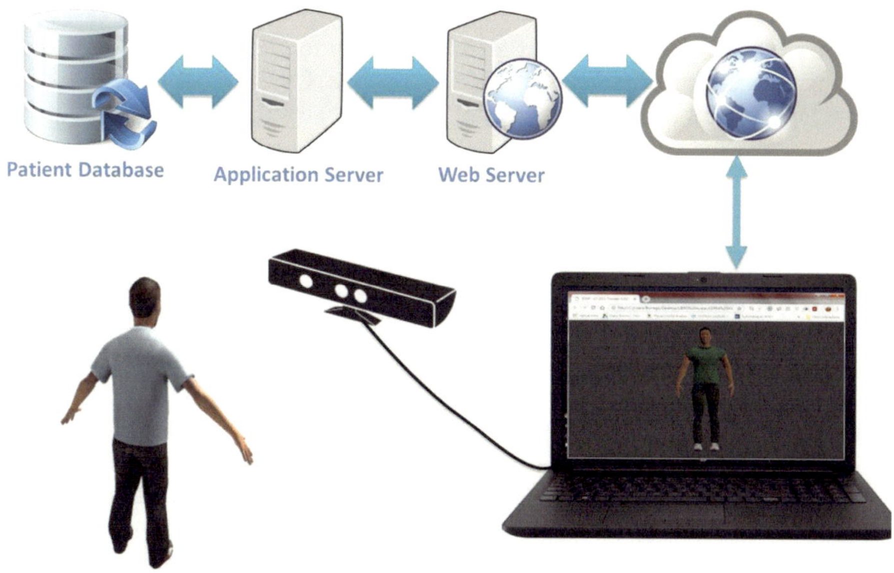

Figure 10.
N-layer architecture of the telerehabilitation platform.

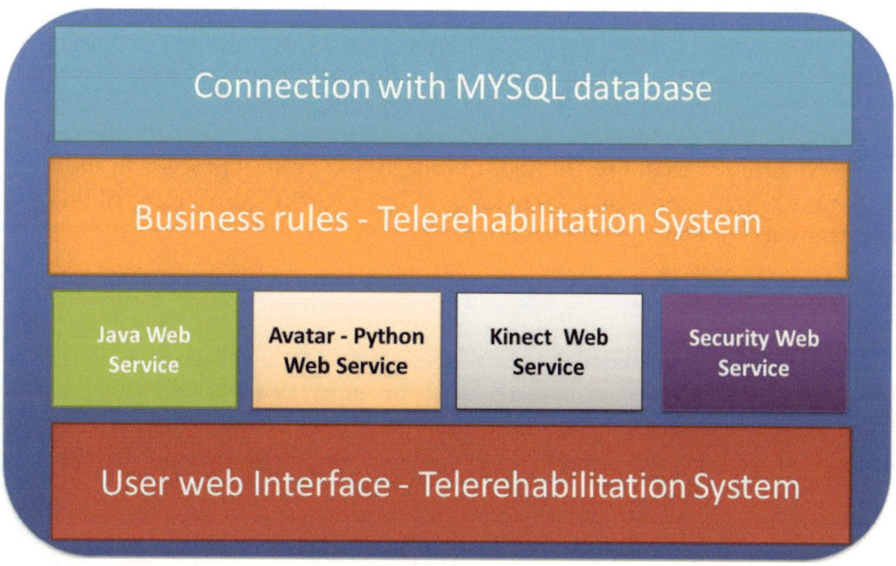

Figure 11.
Telerehabilitation system service-oriented architecture.

	Correctly classified	Incorrectly classified
Well-executed exercise	2100	0
Badly executed exercise	1310	90
Total	**3410**	**90**

Table 2.
Test results in the diffuse model of rehabilitation exercise detection.

In addition, it has been observed in the development of the tests that 18% of the time, the patients perform correctly an exercise with respect to the angle and only 27% do it at an acceptable speed during its execution. On the other hand, the detection time is 0.0045 s while training and 0.002 s in the testing phase.

3. An iterative method to improve the usability of the telerehabilitation system

Usability refers to the degree to which a product can be used to achieve goals in a specific context of use [9]. A software product that has not gone through a process of usability evaluation will not guarantee that users take advantage of the qualities and the benefits of the application. To prevent users from leaving the telerehabilitation platform, it is necessary to carry out exhaustive evaluations of usability.

Several studies have highlighted the main advantages of combining heuristic evaluation and cognitive method for usability assessment [10–13], among them: facility of interaction with the interfaces, immediacy of the response, non-intrusive methods, time or means are not expensive, these tests can be done inside a laboratory, good for the requirements refining, does not involve end users, does not require a fully functional prototype, does not require advance planning, applicable to the stages of design, coding, testing, and implementation of software.

Other studies [12, 14] presented the results of the usability evaluation carried out on the iterative design of the prototypes, obtaining advantages such as facilitating future actions of the end users and improving the learning and development processes. However, the authors said that an online prototype has several drawbacks since it still presents only part of the final version and a limited one in terms of colors and interactive elements. The previous studies do not systematically present the evolution of usability, through an orderly and cyclical process. In addition, these studies do not show that it is possible to improve the use of telerehabilitation platforms without endangering patient safety.

3.1 Experimental design

An experiment was carried out to understand the perceived usability for the ePHoRt platform and to determine a baseline on which to initiate the process of iterative usability improvement of the platform. **Figure 12** shows one on the main interfaces of the platform. The experiment began with 23 participants in an age

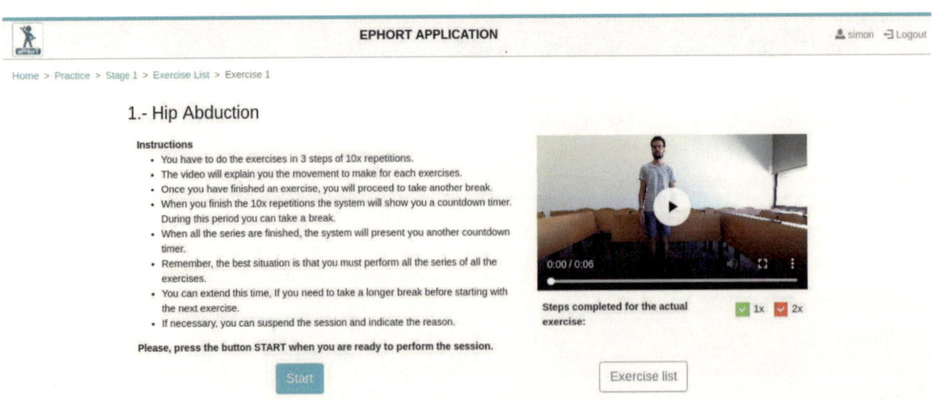

Figure 12.
ePHoRT active exercise interface.

range of 18–24 years old for the first and second iterations, corresponding to the first phase of the experiment. For the second phase, the experiment had 39 participants for the third iteration and 12 participants for the fourth iteration. The age range for these last two iterations was 18–30 years old [15].

3.2 Results

The research results showed improvements in usability through four iterations. Each of the iterations contributed with a list of improvements that were implemented according to the severity level.

In the first iteration, the experts found 39 heuristic violations; these violations were distributed as follows: 12 of high severity, 16 of medium severity, and 11 of low severity. The heuristics with higher incidence and severity were visibility of system status, help and documentation, feedback, and extraordinary users.

In the second iteration, the number of usability problems decreased. However, two atypical cases were presented: (1) increase in the number of usability problems for heuristic "user control and freedom" and heuristic "physical constraint" and (2) the number of usability problems that did not vary for the heuristic "match between the system and the real world" and heuristic "aesthetic and minimalist design."

In the third iteration, 14 mock-ups were designed considering the comments of the previous iterations. In the heuristic evaluation, there were a total of 92 heuristic violations. Experts reported that eight interfaces (57.14%) did not achieve the appropriate feedback for users. Therefore, the platform incurred a clear violation of the heuristic "visibility of system status." In addition, of these eight interfaces, the experts reported the heuristic violation of "help and documentation" on the Login interface and the password reset interface. Finally, experts considered that 42.86% of the interfaces (six) were not flexible or efficient in use.

In the fourth iteration, 17 mock-ups were designed, incorporating the observations from the previous iteration. The experts reported a total of 364 heuristic violations. However, the questionnaire interface had only three low-severity usability problems. This value had been decreasing in severity throughout the evaluation process. The experts assigned greater importance to the following interfaces: questionnaire, acute rehabilitation, active exercise (1/3); acute rehabilitation, active exercise (2/3); acute rehabilitation, active exercise (3/3); and acute rehabilitation, learn (1/5) interfaces.

4. Accessibility of educational resources for the telerehabilitation system

The Web [16] has revolutionized our daily life, becoming the primary source of information, knowledge, consultation, and provision of services and interaction in various areas. Services related to education as well as learning resources are increasing around the world; therefore, it is essential that users, regardless of their disabilities, have accessible learning resources. This study aims to raise awareness of any professional who develops educational applications that apply accessibility standards to generate inclusive and accessible applications. For within the group of possible users, there may be participants with some type of visual disability, such as users with low vision and elderly people. On the other hand, we must emphasize that developing an accessible application does not have to go against an attractive graphical interface, that is, an accessible application does not necessarily have to be "unsightly."

It is convenient to remember that not all visual disabilities are the same and computer management skills also depend on the age of the user, so in the article, these two variables will always be considered. Nowadays, it is necessary to consider the different levels of education, especially for elderly patients and those with disabilities. Therefore, the educational resources of the Tele-habilitation platform must provide instantaneous and ubiquitous access to all types of services and content, including documents and digital resources.

The digital educational resources have become a valuable alternative to support the teaching and learning processes, taking advantage of the possibility of presenting the contents through different multimedia formats. Therefore, it is necessary that educational resources for learning apply accessibility features that allow the interaction of users regardless of their conditions and preferences. This document presents a proposal for the evaluation of the accessibility of multimedia educational resources, where it is suggested to apply the WCAG 2.1 in addition to a series of phases to automatically and manually assess the level of accessibility of the educational resources used in the platform of telerehabilitation of the ePHoRT project.

Accessibility is related to the degree to which people can use or access a service, regardless of their technical, cognitive, or physical abilities [17]. Web accessibility describes methods and theories to make resources, in their multiple forms, more accessible for all people especially for the elderly and people with disabilities. In general, the educational resources of any website or platform must provide universal access, that is, if it includes videos, subtitles must be placed so that the content can be interpreted by people with visual disability or low vision; if people have hearing problems, an audio description should be included, making sure that the resources are inclusive.

The United Nations [18] "Recognizes the importance of access to the physical, social, economic and cultural environment, to health and education and to information and communication, so that persons with disabilities can fully enjoy all human rights and fundamental freedoms."

According to Kurtz et al. [19], the number of people who have undergone surgery for total hip arthroplasty (THA) has increased significantly in the last 10 years, and it is estimated that it will continue to increase.

In line with Ravi et al. [20], THA is a surgery that refers to the replacement of the femoral head and acetabulum of the hip joint. This surgery is usually performed in older adults, due to degenerative joint disease or progressive wear and tear of the joint, and the demographics of patients who decide to undergo THA has become increasingly popular.

In agreement with Salavati et al. [21], the young persons may have higher functional objectives than older persons, which may modify the structuring of rehabilitation protocols. In any of the cases, what is intended after surgery is to calm the pain, restore normal function, and improve the quality of life of people.

In this study, we started with the following question: Are multimedia resources accessible to all users of the telerehabilitation platform?

It is considered an accessible multimedia resource if the content is available to all users, regardless of their disability or application context [22]. It is of vital importance that the educational resources of the platform are accessible even for people who use a screen reader. This research analyzes accessibility problems with multimedia resources, especially those related to video and audio.

According to Rybarczyk et al. [23] in the telerehabilitation platform, learning processes can be oriented in different stages of rehabilitation and include preventive, curative, and maintenance processes.

For the early recovery of the patient on the platform, instructions are included on the general consequences of the procedures and their likely risks, so it is intended to guide the patient through the rehabilitation process at all stages. Proper guidance can help the patient make the right movements to reinforce the safety of functional tasks and motivate the patient to complete the rehabilitation program. Considering that the patient should perform the exercises in a standing position and at a certain distance from the computer, inclusive resources are proposed to guide the patient in the learning process. One of the main elements that have proven to be useful and efficient in education as a means of transmitting and strengthening knowledge is the implementation of multimedia teaching materials, including the use of videos, audios, and PDF files, which constitute an excellent support material. Conforming to Acosta-Vargas et al. [24], the method used to assess access to educational resources consists of identifying the type of resource, reviewing access barriers to the resource according to WCAG 2.1, combining automatic and manual methods to assess the accessibility of resources, recording identified barriers in a spreadsheet, analyzing the results, and finally suggesting possible recommendations.

4.1 Accessibility

Baruch et al. [25] indicate that multimedia accessibility policies propose that "All multimedia elements such as audio or video, produced or published must be accessible at the time of publication." Multimedia accessibility proposes a simple text transcription, so that it is necessary to place a transcript in audio-only recordings, to meet all the success criteria suggested by WCAG 2.1. On the other hand, multimedia resources according to the World Wide Web Consortium (W3C) [26] include texts, images, graphics, animations, video, and sound to present or communicate specific information. Consequently, to cover all the parameters that intervene in the accessibility of educational resources, it is necessary to evaluate a set of dependent components such as human factors, in this case all the users of the telerehabilitation platform are considered, including users with special needs, technological factors to provide accessibility, and user interaction with the device in the environment of the platform, which include criteria to favor accessibility with the indicated components. ISO/IEC 40500: 2012 [27] is equivalent to the Web Content Accessibility Guidelines 2.0 (WCAG 2.0), is related to the Web Content Accessibility Guidelines 2.1 (WCAG 2.1) which consists of 4 principles, 13 guidelines, and 76 compliance criteria (success), plus an undetermined number of sufficient techniques and counseling techniques.

The four principles are the same as those contained in WCAG 2.0:

- Principle 1—Perceptibility: information and user interface components should be presented to users in the way they can be perceived. It has 4 guidelines and 29 compliance criteria.

- Principle 2—Operability: the user interface and the navigation components must be operable. It has 5 guidelines and 29 compliance criteria.

- Principle 3—Comprehensibility: the information and management of the user interface must be understandable. It has 3 guidelines and 17 compliance criteria.

- Principle 4—Robustness: the content must be robust enough to be based on its interpretation by a wide variety of user agents, including assistive technologies. It has one guideline and three compliance criteria.

4.2 Method

In March 2012, Web Accessibility Initiative (WAI) published the Methodology of Website Accessibility Conformance Evaluation Methodology (WCAG-EM) 1.0. In 2014, a new version was published [28]. The WCAG-EM methodology allows

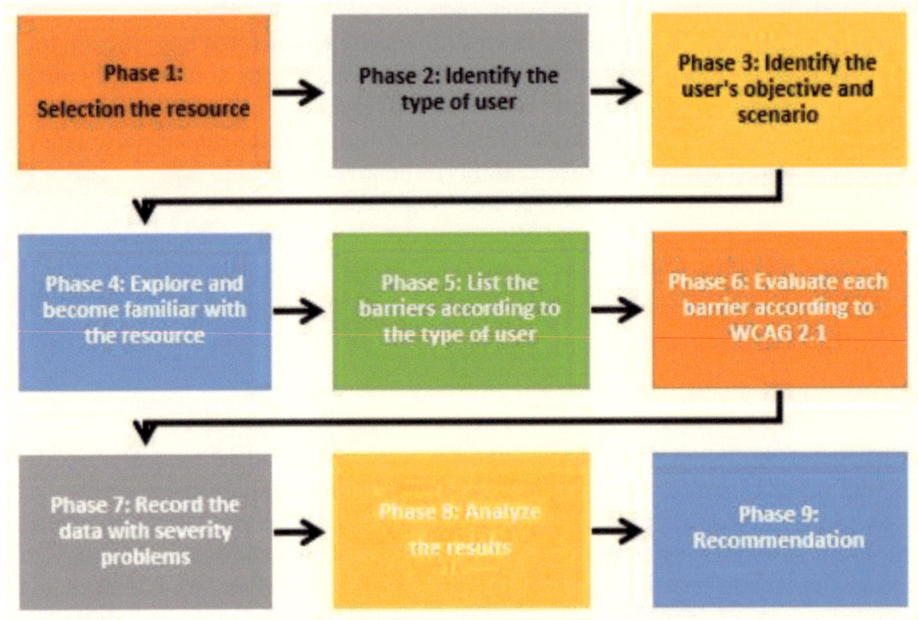

Figure 13.
Evaluation of multimedia resources.

determining if the contents of the websites are evaluated to comply with the WCAG 2.1 accessibility guidelines or not. In this research the WCAG-EM 1.0 was applied. In this case, it was used to apply the evaluation of multimedia resources specifically to the videos. It consists of five sequential phases, as shown in **Figure 13**.

Phase 1: Selection of the resource. In this phase, the educational resource to be evaluated is selected. For this study, the video located on the telerehabilitation platform was selected. **Figure 14** shows a screenshot; it is observed that the patient performs rehabilitation exercises. It should be noted that this resource is part of the patient education section and the educational resources will be hosted on the platform located at http://telerehabilitation.udla.edu.ec/learning/resource/2/media/1.

Phase 2: Identify the type of user. In this phase, the type of users is defined; for our case we will focus on older people who have age-related disabilities [29]; this may affect the way they use the web, like first, the reduction of the vision that includes a sensitivity reduced to the contrast, the perception of the color, and the near approach. This makes difficult the reading of the web pages. Second is the reduction of physical capacity including dexterity. This makes it difficult to use the mouse and click on small targets. Third is the difficulty of listening, including the difficulty to hear sharp sounds and separate sounds. This makes it difficult to listen to podcasts and other audio, especially when there is background music. Fourth, cognitive ability includes short-term memory reduction, difficulty concentrating, and being easily distracted, which makes it difficult to track browsing and online tasks. These problems are related to the accessibility needs of people with disabilities. Therefore, websites, applications, and tools that are accessible to people with disabilities are also more accessible to older users.

Phase 3: Identify the user's real scenario. In this phase, it is determined what the patient wants to learn in the telerehabilitation platform so that the educational resource adequately explains the process so that the patient learns and reinforces his learning.

Phase 4: Explore and become familiar with the resource. In this phase, we review the resource format for our case study and review the video format, size, and

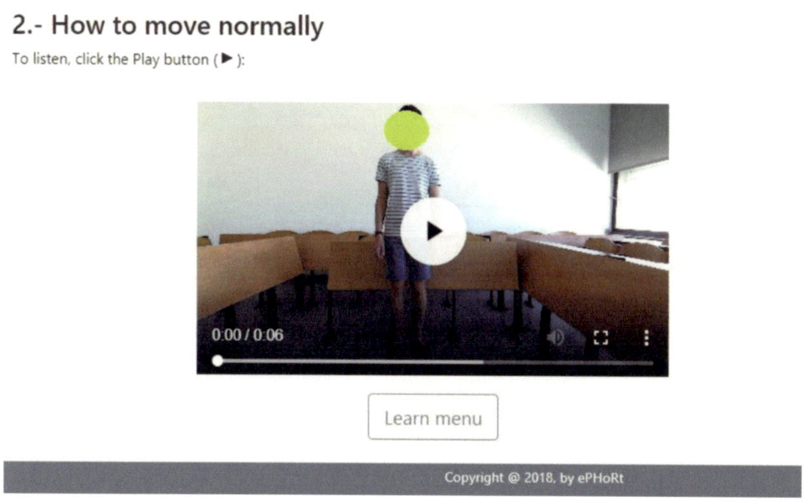

Figure 14.
Screenshot of the resource to evaluate.

duration. This information is relevant to review with the Photosensitive Epilepsy Analysis Tool[1] (PEAT) [30] of the University of Wisconsin Trace Center. It is required that the video is in Audio Video Interleave (AVI) format.

Table 3 records the results obtained in the evaluation with PEAT. It contains the video identifier, length of material, luminance flash failures, red flash failures, extended flash warnings, result status, and percentage.

Phase 5: List the barriers according to the type of user. In this phase, the possible barriers that the user can find in the resource are established, such as the keyboard compatibility, the colors with good contrast, the design and bright design, the text of voice, extensive links, buttons and controls, video descriptions, customizable text, speech recognition, understandable content, notifications and comments, and selection to different language types. That relates to the WCAG 2.1 success criteria detailed in **Table 4**.

Phase 6: Evaluate each barrier according to WCAG 2.1. In this phase, the criteria of success are evaluated manually according to WCAG 2.1. About the principle of perceptible [31], the Guideline 1.2 related to time-based media. According to the criterion of success 1.2.1, either only audio or only prerecorded video (Level A), it is necessary to provide an alternative that describes the content of the prerecorded video, for example, placing an audio track. Criteria of success 1.2.2 subtitles

URL	Description	Standard	Success criterion	Fr	Lm	Rs	Lff	Rff	Efw
http://telerehabilitation.udla.edu.ec/learning/resource/2/media/1	Patient in the process of learning exercises on the telerehabilitation platform	WCAG 2.1	2.3	25	00:06.19	P	0	0	0

Fr = frame rate, Lm = length of material, Rs = result status, Lff = luminance flash failures, Rff = red flash failures, Efw = extended flash warnings, P = passed

Table 3.
Evaluation with the photosensitive epilepsy analysis tool.

[1] http://trace.umd.edu/peat

Success criterion	Level	Comply
1.2.1 Audio-only and video-only (prerecorded)	A	1
1.2.2 Captions (prerecorded)	A	0
1.2.3 Audio description or media alternative (prerecorded)	A	0
1.2.4 Captions (live)	AA	0
1.2.5 Audio description (prerecorded)	AA	0
1.2.6 Sign language (prerecorded)	AAA	0
1.2.7 Extended audio description (prerecorded)	AAA	0
1.2.8 Media alternative (prerecorded)	AAA	0
1.2.9 Audio-only (live)	AAA	0

Table 4.
Manual evaluation of the video resource.

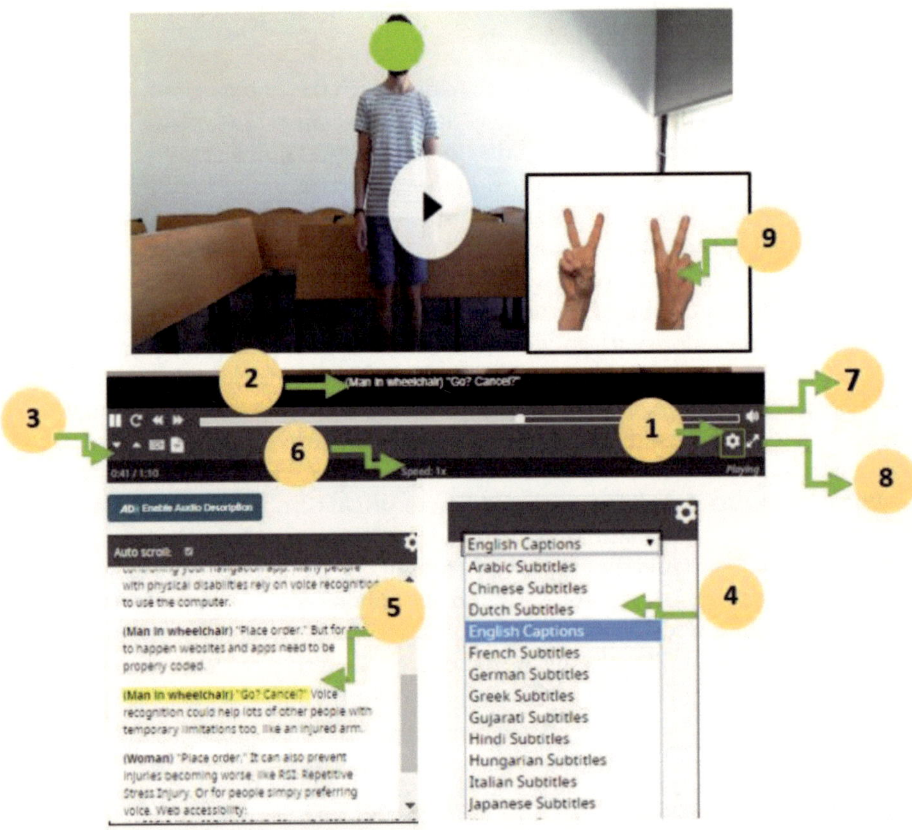

Figure 15.
Recommendations for the creation of accessible videos.

(Level A) are as follows: subtitles are provided for all prerecorded audio content in synchronized media, except when the media are an alternative media for text and are clearly labeled as such. The criterion of success 1.2.3 related to the description of audio or alternative of prerecorded media (Level A). It suggests that an alternative is provided for synchronized media, except when the medium is a multimedia alternative to the text and is clearly labeled as such. Success criteria 1.2.4 subtitles (live) (Level AA) are as follows: subtitles are provided for all live audio content in synchronized media. Success criterion 1.2.5, which refers to the description of prerecorded audio (Level AA), provides audio description for all prerecorded video content in synchronized media. Success criterion 1.2.6 sign language (level AAA) provides sign language interpretation for all prerecorded audio content in synchronized media. Success criterion 1.2.7 related to having an extended audio description for all prerecorded video content (Level AAA) to use when the foreground audio is insufficient to convey the meaning of the video. Success criterion 1.2.8 on the prerecorded media alternative (Level AAA) provides an alternative for time-based media for all prerecorded synchronized media and for all prerecorded video media only. Finally, success criterion 1.2.9 audio only (Level AAA) provides an alternative for time-based media that presents equivalent information for live audio-only content on media only. **Table 2** shows the data of the manually evaluated video resource. It contains the success criterion of WCAG 2.1 of the perceptible principle, level, and compliance that indicate whether it meets the success criteria, where 1 indicates that it meets and 0 indicates that it does not comply.

Phase 7: Record the data with severity problems. In this phase, the results are recorded in a spreadsheet; in this case, Microsoft Excel was used. The data record and the analysis of the results to replicate the research are available in the Mendeley dataset.[2]

Phase 8: Analyze the results. In this phase, the authors used Microsoft Excel statistical graphs. The dispersion graph was applied with the trend line to analyze the value of R between the success criteria and compliance with the WCAG 2.1.

Phase 9: Recommendation. In this phase, some recommendations are suggested so that the video resource is accessible and inclusive, according to WCAG 2.1. In **Figure 15** according to the numbering, it is described what it should contain in each element so that the video resource is more inclusive and accessible. See details below:

1. Preferences. In this option, it should allow the configuration of subtitles, descriptions, keyboard, and transcription.

2. Show the subtitle settings. In this case, it should include the options to configure according to the preference of users such as position, font, font size, text color, background, and opacity.

3. Video speed, subtitles, and audio in the application. The user should have the option to customize the speed of the video, subtitles, and audio according to the user's preference and disability.

4. Language. In this option, the user could customize and choose the language for the audio description and subtitles. This option should allow moving the window to the position you want the user to.

5. Audio description preferences. In this option, the media player must allow the configuration of the audio description format in several ways so that it is displayed in the highlighted form of the color the user wishes while the video is presented. In addition, it is vital to include the option of automatic video pause and the option to make the description visible. On the other hand, it is essential to include keyboard preferences using keyboard shortcuts. This option should allow moving the window to the position you want the user to.

[2] http://dx.doi.org/10.17632/tjf47zxmv2.1

6. Visualize the speed of the video. In this option, the user can visualize the speed in the video according to the configured speed.

7. Volume. In this option, the user can configure the volume of the audio.

8. Screen. In this option, the user can view the video in full screen.

9. Sign language. In this option, you can include a screen with a description of it in sign language.

5. Results

In the evaluation of the accessibility of an educational resource, it is vital to combine the automatic tools with manual evaluation. In this case, for the video, a resource is not yet known as an automatic tool that performs the evaluation at 100%. In the automatic evaluation, the tool PEAT was applied, which helps to identify the luminance flaw faults, the red flashing faults, and the extended flashing warnings that would affect users with epilepsy. According to the PEAT report, it is observed that it overcomes the problem.

The evaluation was complemented with a manual analysis when considering the possible barriers for the users of the telerehabilitation platform. The results are detailed in **Table 4**.

In **Figure 16**, it is observed that the video does not comply with the WCAG 2.1 guidelines, that is, it is not inclusive. When applying the correlation between the success criteria and compliance, the coefficient is −0.5. This implies that the correlation is negative and moderate. Failures are related to the absence to configure user preferences by including keyboard compatibility, colors with good contrast, bright design, text to speech, links, buttons and controls, video subtitles, customizable text, speech recognition, understandable content, notifications, and comments.

The results of this study show that the multimedia resource evaluated did not reach an acceptable level of accessibility. Therefore, it is necessary to correct the

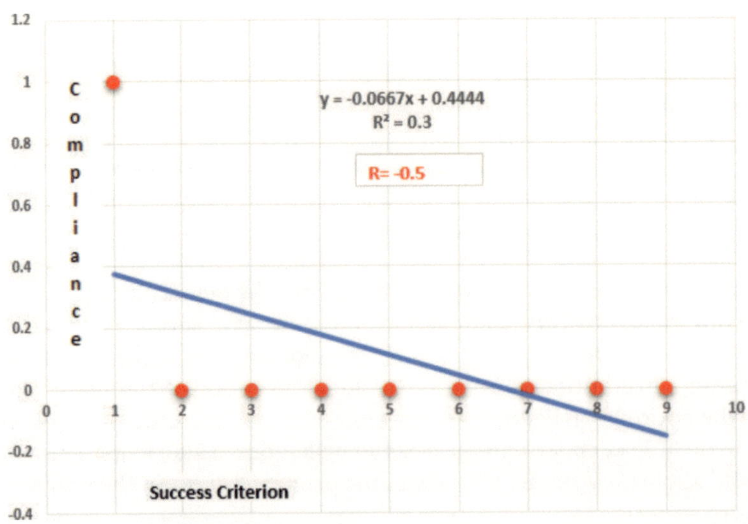

Figure 16.
Analysis of success criteria vs. compliance.

faults to comply with the level of accessibility recommended by the W3C. It is necessary to include accessibility measures in the development of educational materials through the application of a checklist to correct the problems identified. The results obtained in the evaluation can serve as a starting point to implement future video resources considering WCAG 2.1.

The recommendations suggested in phase 9 can provide ideas on how to develop and create educational videos to make them more accessible and inclusive. This research can serve as base information for future projects with a more significant number of educational resources. Future research may propose new methods to evaluate multimedia resources. With respect to the videos and sound recordings, in both cases, a transcription of the dialogues, a description of the sounds, and control of the reproduction speed must be provided. However, the inappropriate use of multimedia elements may cause a barrier to user access.

6. Conclusions

The application of the fuzzy logic technique in a telerehabilitation platform allowed identifying correct and incorrect movements in the execution of rehabilitation exercises of patients after hip surgery. The main contributions of the proposed fuzzy detection algorithm are flexibility, tolerance with inaccuracy, and the ability to identify features that best predict different points of movement.

The design of avatars allowed the digital representations of the patient's movements captured with Microsoft's Kinect. The main contributions are to monitor exercises in real time, to identify the recovery progress of patients, to provide medical information to physiotherapeutic, and to facilitate an engaging experience for patients.

The limitation that we found in the implemented model is that it was very useful for exercises that are performed standing; however there are exercises that the patient performs lying down, in which Kinect was not able to capture patient's movements, and it is recommended for future work to use other type of sensors.

The web application of a diffuse 3D model for the detection of rehabilitation exercises after a hip surgery is systematically related to the usability and accessibility of the telerehabilitation system in search of achieving inclusive websites that display correctly on any device.

The method applied in improving the usability and accessibility of educational resources for the telerehabilitation system is very important since access to the Internet is a growing trend. This project addressed the importance of applying the principles specified in WCAG 2.1 to develop accessible resources. The development and execution of this project can serve as a starting point to develop targeted strategies to raise awareness about the importance of the stages of design of a website or educational resources, where the accessibility guidelines and criteria must be applied in order to achieve equal access to information for all people.

Finally, the system has limitations since it is not possible to guarantee for a web page or educational resource to be accessible for all types of users with disabilities or to comply with all accessibility standards.

Acknowledgements

This research has been partially supported by the *Consorcio Ecuatoriano para el Desarrollo de Internet Avanzado (CEDIA),* Grant CEPRA-XI-2017-2115.

Author details

Patricia Acosta-Vargas[1], Janio Jadán-Guerrero[2], Cesar Guevara[2], Sandra Sanchez-Gordon[3]* and Tania Calle-Jimenez[3]

1 Intelligent and Interactive Systems Lab, Universidad de Las Américas, Quito, Ecuador

2 Universidad Tecnológica Indoamérica, Quito, Ecuador

3 Department of Informatics and Computer Science, Escuela Politécnica Nacional, Quito, Ecuador

*Address all correspondence to: sandra.sanchez@epn.edu.ec

References

[1] Rautaray S, Agrawal A. Vision based hand gesture recognition for human computer interaction: A survey. Artificial Intelligence Review. 2015;**43**(1):1-54

[2] Ichim A, Bouaziz S, Pauly M. Dynamic 3D avatar creation from hand-held video input. ACM Transactions on Graphics. 2015;**34**(4):45:1-45:14

[3] Pavone E, Tieri G, Rizza G, Tidoni E, Grisoni L, Aglioti S. Embodying others in immersive virtual reality: Electro-cortical signatures of monitoring the errors in the actions of an avatar seen from a first-person perspective. The Journal of Neuroscience. 2016;**36**(2):268-279

[4] Belal S, Taktak A, Nevill A, Spencer S. A fuzzy system for detecting distorted plethysmogram pulses in neonates and paediatric patients. Physiological Measurement. 2001;**22**(2):397-412

[5] Guevara C, Jadán-Guerrero J, Rybarczyk Y, Acosta-Vargas P, Esparza W, González M, et al. A real-time algorithm for movement assessment using fuzzy logic of hip arthroplasty patients. In: Advances in Intelligent Systems and Computing. Vol. 781. Cham: Springer; 2019. pp. 265-273

[6] Han J, Shao L, Xu D, Shotton J. Enhanced computer vision with Microsoft Kinect sensor: A review. IEEE Transactions on Cybernetics. 2013;**43**(5):1318-1334

[7] Sastry S. Intelligent Control. CRC Press; 2018

[8] Suganthi L, Iniyan S, Samuel A. Applications of fuzzy logic in renewable energy systems—A review. Renewable and Sustainable Energy Reviews. 2015;**48**:585-607

[9] International Organization for Standardization. ISO 9241-11—Ergonomics of human system interaction. 2018

[10] Kushniruk A, Monkman H, Tuden D, Bellwood P, Borycki E. Integrating heuristic evaluation with cognitive walkthrough: Development of a hybrid usability inspection method. In: Studies in Health Technology and Informatics. Vol. 208. 2015. pp. 221-225

[11] Xiao L, Yan X, Emery A. Design and evaluation of web interfaces for informal care providers in senior monitoring. In: Proceedings of the 76th ASIS&T Annual Meeting: Beyond the Cloud: Rethinking Information Boundaries; 2013

[12] Gulati A, Sanjay K. Critical analysis on usability evaluation techniques. International Journal of Engineering Science and Technology (IJEST). 2012;**4**

[13] Lim C, Hae-Deok S, Lee Y. Improving the usability of the user interface for a digital textbook platform for elementary-school students. Educational Technology Research Development. 2012;**60**:159-173

[14] Quinones D, Rusu C. How to develop usability heuristics: A systematic literature review. Computer Standards and Interfaces. 2017;**53**:89-122

[15] Pilco H, Sanchez-Gordon S, Calle-Jimenez T, Rybarczyk Y, Jadán J, Villarreal S, et al. Analysis and improvement of the usability of a tele-rehabilitation platform for hip surgery patients. In: Advances in Intelligent Systems and Computing. Vol. 781. Cham: Springer; 2019. pp. 197-209

[16] Acosta-Vargas P, Acosta T, Lujan-Mora S. Challenges to assess accessibility in higher education websites: A comparative study of

Latin-America universities. IEEE Access. 2018;**6**:36500-36508

[17] Acosta-Vargas P, Luján-Mora S, Acosta T, Salvador-Ullauri L. Toward a combined method for evaluation of web accessibility. In: Advances in Intelligent Systems and Computing. Vol. 721. Cham: Springer; 2018. pp. 602-613

[18] United Nations. Convention on the rights of persons with disabilities. Treaty Series. 2006;**2515**(3)

[19] Kurtz S, Ong K, Lau E, Bozic K. Impact of the economic downturn on total joint replacement demand in the United States: Updated projections to 2021. Journal of Bone and Joint Surgery. American. 2014;**96**(8):624-630

[20] Ravi B, Croxford R, Reichmann W, Losina E, Katz J, Hawker G. The changing demographics of total joint arthroplasty recipients in the United States and Ontario from 2001 to 2007. Best Practice & Research. Clinical Rheumatology. 2012;**26**(5):637-647

[21] Salavati A et al. Optimal FDG PET/CT volumetric parameters for risk stratification in patients with locally advanced non-small cell lung cancer: results from the ACRIN 6668/RTOG 0235 trial. European Journal of Nuclear Medicine and Molecular Imaging. 2017;**44**(12):1969-1983

[22] Brady E, Zhong Y, Bigham J. Creating accessible PDFs for conference proceedings. In: Proc. 12th Web All Conf. - W4A '15. 2015. pp. 1-4

[23] Rybarczyk Y, Deters J, Gonzalo A, Esparza D, Gonzalez M, Villarreal S, et al. Recognition of physiotherapeutic exercises through DTW and low-cost vision-based motion capture. In: Advances in Human Factors and Systems Interaction. Vol. 592. Cham: Springer; 2017. pp. 348-360

[24] Acosta-Vargas P, Esparza W, Rybarczyk Y, González M, Villarreal S, Jadán J, et al. Educational resources accessible on the tele-rehabilitation platform. In: Advances in Human Factors and Systems Interaction. Vol. 781. Cham: Springer; 2019. pp. 210-220

[25] Baruch H, Ehrlich J, Yaffe A. Splinting—A review of the literature. Refuat Hapeh Vehashinayim. 2001;**18**(1):29-40

[26] World Wide Web Consortium. Multimedia Accessibility FAQ. 2016. Available from: https://www.w3.org/2008/06/video-notes [Accessed: 11-Nov-2018]

[27] International Standards Organization. ISO/IEC 40500:2012 Information technology—W3C Web Content Accessibility Guidelines (WCAG) 2.0. 2012. Available online: https://www.w3.org/TR/WCAG20/. 2008. [Accessed: 11-Nov-2018]

[28] World Wide Web Consortium. Website Accessibility Conformance Evaluation Methodology (WCAG-EM) 1.0. 2014. Available online: https://www.w3.org/TR/WCAG-EM/ [Accessed: 11-Nov-2018]

[29] World Wide Web Consortium. Web accessibility perspectives: Explore the impact and benefits for everyone—Web Accessibility Initiative (WAI). Available online: https://w3c.github.io/wai-website/perspective-videos/. 2018. [Accessed: 11-Nov-2018]

[30] World Wide Web Consortium. Web Accessibility Evaluation Tools List. 2018. Available online: https://www.w3.org/WAI/ER/tools/?q=mobile-application. [Accessed: 11-Nov-2018]

[31] World Wide Web Consortium. Web Content Accessibility Guidelines (WCAG) 2.1. 2018. Available online: https://www.w3.org/TR/WCAG21/

Chapter 6

MedBike: Virtual Reality for Remote Cardiac Rehabilitation

Pierre Boulanger, William Mott, Stephanie Schaeffer, Peter W. Wood, Raj Padwal and Paolo Raggi

Abstract

Exercise-based cardiac rehabilitation (exCR) is a key element of a multidisciplinary cardiac rehabilitation program towards the care of patients with acute or chronic cardiac disease. Many studies have shown that patient's adherence to these programs is low despite evidence that such programs can improve outcomes and critical cardiac event reduction. New strategies to improve adherence to exCR programs are now being tested using non-hospital solutions that relies on VR gaming technologies. This paper presents such a system called MedBike which allows patients to perform an exCR program at home while being monitored in real-time by a remote clinician. The paper describes the technical aspects of the system, its pros and cons, various gamification strategies, and a recent usability study.

Keywords: virtual reality, haptics, telemonitoring, cardiac rehabilitation

1. Introduction

Exercise-based cardiac rehabilitation (exCR) is a key component of a multidisciplinary cardiac rehabilitation program. Advances in medical and surgical cardiac treatments have improved the outcome for patients with acute or chronic cardiac diseases. In addition to those treatments, cardiac rehabilitation can provide great improvements to patient's outcome by reducing cardiovascular mortality, rehospitalization, and improving patient's quality of life [1]. Patient's adherence to these programs is low despite evidence that such programs can improve outcomes and reduce critical cardiac events. These low adherence rates have been shown to be between 15 and 30% [2–4]. A recent analysis of a large United States study (n = 74, 798) have shown that only 5.4% of eligible patients finished an exCR program [5]. Adherence to an exCR is critical as non-participants exhibit a 30% lower survival rate compare to patient's following a complete rehabilitation program [6].

Many factors improving the adherence to an exCR program have been identified. These factors include lack of physician endorsement, traveling distance from the patient's home to the hospital, lack of transportation, cost (e.g., parking fees), low self-motivation, poor social support, low self-esteem, fear of precipitating a cardiac event, and lack of enjoyment [4–9]. If one could improve the enjoyment of exCR activities using VR gaming technologies, one could increase program adherence as patients who have a positive view of exercise are more likely to continue [10, 11]. A recent study by Taylor et al. [12] reported that simply placing exCR in a home was not enough to improve program compliance. There are increasing interests in exploring how VR gaming technology can improve CR participation by decentralizing the exCR process, increasing accessibility to rehabilitation, and increasing its comfort and enjoyment. This approach follows a recommendation by the American Heart Association's that internet-based techniques can be used to improve cardiac rehabilitation for both patients and healthcare providers [13].

Cardiac rehabilitation therapy is a long-term and tedious treatment. In recent years, virtual reality (VR) technologies have reduced in price and increased in visual quality and is now being used for many medical applications such as: therapies in CR [14], pain reduction [15, 16], stress reduction and skill training [17], telerehabilitation [18], and education [19]. Virtual rehabilitation applications using gaming technologies to improve interests to a rehabilitation program and the ability for a therapist to adapt a patient specific exercise program locally or remotely using the internet is currently being explored. By using VR technologies, a therapist can set a variety of controlled stimuli, monitor patients' responses during the exercise program, and offer clinical assessment and options [20, 21]. Using these VR systems, patients are immersed in a virtual environment, allowing them to perform safely physical activities [22]. Research [23] in the human physiological response to immersive VR systems was able to demonstrate that a significant increase in cycling time, distance, and caloric expenditure can be observed in healthy seniors and

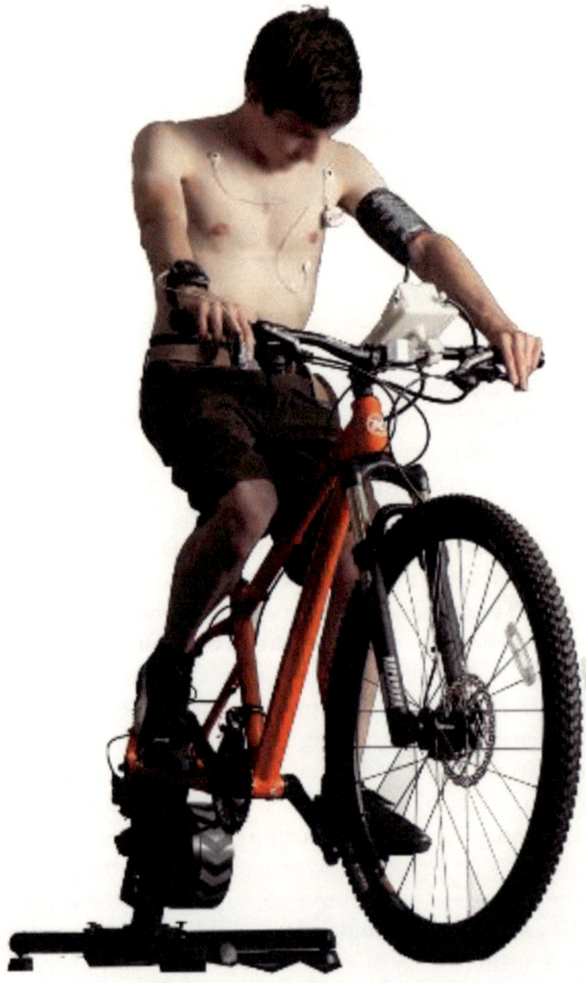

Figure 1.
MedBike the VR-based telemonitored exercise cardiac rehabilitation system.

juniors using such systems. A review on how VR system can help enhance exercise performance, enjoyment, and dissociation can be found in [24].

This paper describes the MedBike cardiac rehabilitation system (see **Figure 1**) which consists of a mountain bike mounted on a wirelessly controlled programmable resistance machine connected to a Unity 3D based VR game engine. Using this system patients can cycle through a virtual landscape where the bicycle resistance is modulated by the virtual world terrain and maximum/minimum forces set by a clinician. During the exercise program, the patients are monitored remotely by an exCR clinician in real-time using wireless biometric sensors (ECG, blood pressure, and pulse oximetry) and a bidirectional audio-video Internet connection. Section 2 describes the basic element of the MedBike system design specifications and implementation. Section 3 describes our current attempt to improve adherence to exCR programs through VR gamification. Section 4 describes MedBike effectiveness to improve exCR from a usability, adherence, and fitness point-of-view. We then conclude by discussing the pros and cons of the system.

2. MedBike system overview

Numerous designs for instrumented bikes have been proposed in the literature and in industry; additionally, a number of patents have also been awarded. The closest to our system, in which a VR controllable resistance system was developed for a cardio fitness application was proposed in [25, 26]. Commercial virtual reality cycling systems that use VR and instrumented bicycles have appeared on the market. The Italian company Widerun [27] offers clients to connect a normal bike to their resistance device, put on a VR headset, and cycle across a virtual terrain representing world-class cycling circuits. Their system can provide variable resistance based on the in-game environment. The overall visual quality is good but is not equal to the image quality produced by Unity 3D game engine. Their system uses a Head Mounted Displays (HMD) for immersion but as demonstrated in our lab, HMD are highly disorientating which may result in falls. Their system also does not provide free steering/breaking capabilities. The American company Zwift [28] is the one that closely resembles the VR aspects of MedBike. Contrary to our system, Zwift's worlds are static and not very engaging and cannot be modified easily for gamification. Zwift's graphics rendering suffers from many visual anomalies like aliasing and poor level of details via pop-up. Most of these commercial systems target the pro-cycling niche market focusing mainly on exercise performance and training, not medical applications. Most are them are dedicated cycling systems and cannot be easily modified for gamification. None of these systems offers patient sensor-based telemonitoring.

Following numerous discussions with CR clinicians, we came up with design specifications for the system that are as follows:

- Privacy and data transmission integrity are critical;
- VR experience does not need to be stereo or use HMDs because of concerns for patient's balance and the loss of awareness of his/her environment;
- All patient's telemetry sensors should be medical grade;
- Telemetry sensors must be easy to install by the patient;
- Patient's interface must be intuitive and must be easy to use and should not necessitate computer technical knowledge;

- The patient system must be able to work on public internet services with bandwidth not exceeding 5 Mbps;
- A patient should be able to see animated avatars of other patients connected to the system;
- Clinician should be able to monitor six patients at a time which include:
    - Real-time access to patient's vital signs, current power produced, cadence, etc.;
    - Access to data from previous MedBike sessions, including from player sessions (sessions completed individually without clinician);
    - Patient's medical records;
    - Secure video conferencing with each patient;
    - Ability to specify exercise parameters such as target power and cadence ranges that must be achieved;
    - Ability to record medical notes and performance of the patient during a session.

2.1 Patient's VR system

One can see in **Figure 2** the patient's MedBike hardware configuration. The system consists of a mountain bike mounted on a wirelessly controlled resistance machine (KICKR) from Wahoo Inc. The resistance machine is connected to the patient's PC using an ANT+ interface. The bike is also instrumented with a professional wireless (ANT+) cadence sensor. In addition, a steering sensor composed of a rotary encoder is mounted on the handle bar, digitized by a Phidgets board and connected by USB to the graphic PC. The bike is also instrumented by an Android tablet mounted on the handle bar which is responsible for collecting the vital sign sensors (ECG, Oximeter, Blood Pressure meter) using Bluetooth (**Figure 3**). The tablet is also used as the main interface for the patient initiating authentication, selecting and modifying menu items, and controlling bike system states. The high-end graphic control PC is a machine that renders Unity 3D world which is

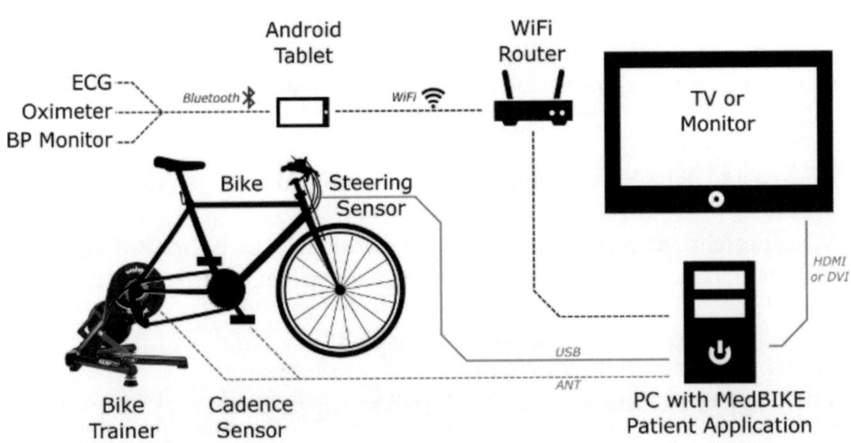

Figure 2.
MedBike patient hardware.

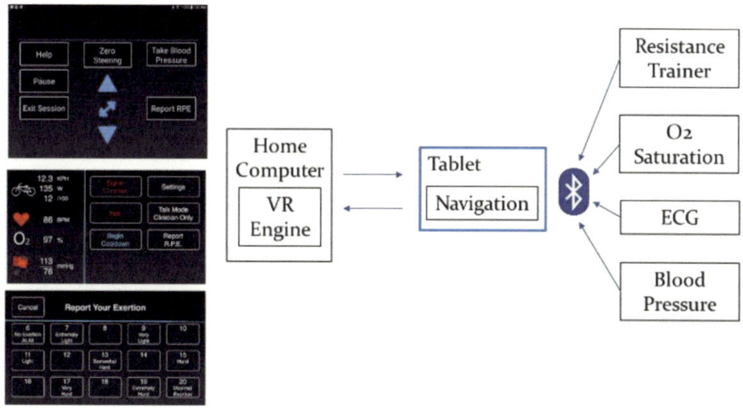

Figure 3.
Android tablet for interface and data HUB.

synchronized with the bike sensors and the training parameters specified by the clinician. This computer system is used as a data transmission HUB (See **Figure 4**) and is responsible to:

- Render the Unity 3D world based on bike sensor data (see **Figure 5**);
- Control the bike programmable resistance machine using the virtual world terrain and resistance limits specified by the clinician;
- Establish encrypted audio/video connection between the clinician and the patient using WebRTC;
- Perform medical data transmission to the patient's data using standard encryption algorithm;
- Save patient information to a cloud-based server using Django application and a MySQL database;
- Receive encrypted clinician information that set the minimum and maximum cadence as well as the power ranges a patient should achieve during his/her training;
- Update, using the internet, other cyclist avatar locations and status if the system is in multi-player mode.

2.2 Clinician's telemonitoring system

On the clinician side, the system is based on a high-end PC where all the information from up to six patients can be displayed and analyzed (see **Figures 6** and **7**). The session starts by first establishing patient and clinician authentication credentials with the MedBike server. Once established, each patient is attributed an encryption key to encode the information transmitted during the session.

For each patient, the clinician set a unique exercise program using an exercise program editor. Each patient-specific exercise program can have an arbitrary number of stages with different lengths and target power outputs. Typically, these exercise programs include a warm-up, exercise, and cool-down stages. Other programs can also be specified such as high-intensity interval training (HIIT) parameters. These exercise programs include:

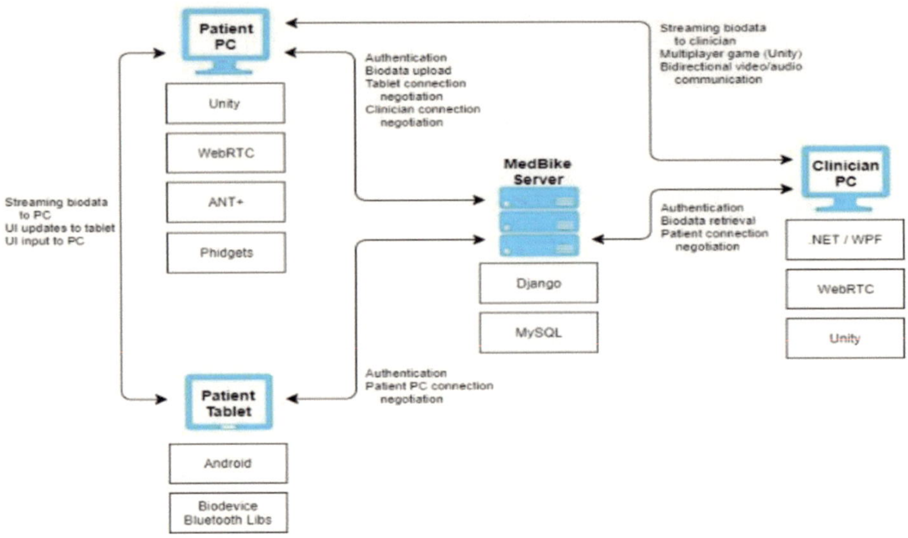

Figure 4.
MedBike system dataflow.

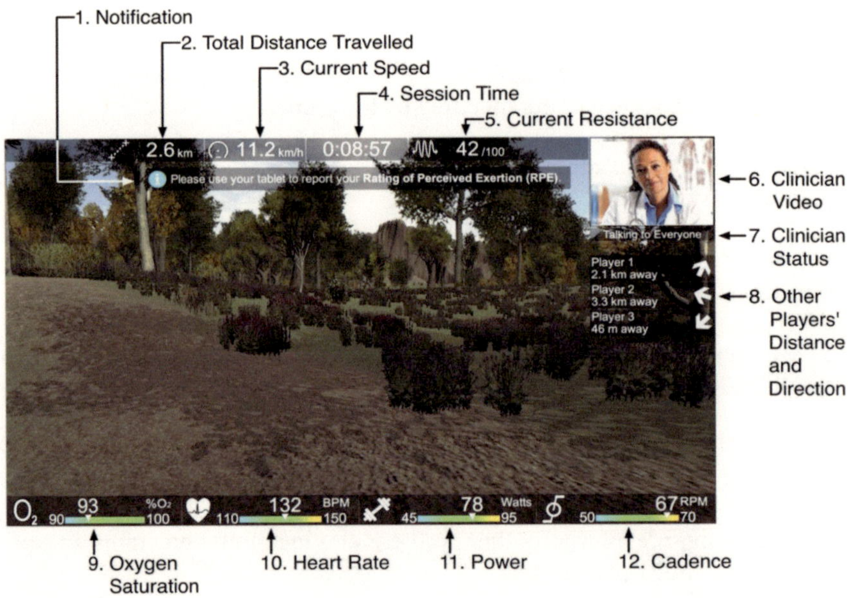

Figure 5.
Patient's VR display.

Global values: These values apply to all stages of the exercise prescription.

- Target resistances: It is specified by the minimum and maximum resistance allowed for the bike trainer to use. These values range from 0 (no resistance) to 100 (full resistance).
- Rate of perceived exertion (RPE) Scale and Target RPE: The RPE scale to use and the optimal range of RPE values. Optimal values specified here will appear in green on patient's tablets, except for the pediatric scale, which has its own color coding. Default optimal values for the adult scale are between 11 and 15.

- Weekly goal: This is the recommended number of single player exercise sessions per week.
- Target oxygen saturation: Optionally, a target minimum oxygen saturation value can be specified.

Per-Stage Values: These values define the various exercise stages in the prescription. Stages can be added, removed, and their position adjusted. Each stage includes the following values:

- Stage Name: the name of the stage (e.g., warm-up, exercise, etc.).
- Stage Duration: the length of the stage, in minutes and seconds.
- Target Power: the target power in Watts for this stage. These values are used to adjust the difficulty of the bicycling experience for the patient. If the power requirements input here are high, then the patient will be given a higher resistance to work against to increase their power output.
- Target Cadence: optionally, a target cadence in RPM.
- Target Heart Rate: specify minimum and maximum heart rate targets for the patient.
- RPE Prompts: specified, the system can automatically prompt patients for RPE at predetermined times.
- Blood pressure (BP) measurements: if specified, the system can automatically initiate a blood pressure measurement after a certain percentage of the stage is completed.

The system generates a post session report which was developed in partnership with cardiac rehabilitation clinicians, to best meet there clinical reporting requirements. The system also allows the clinician access to past session reports. A typical session report (which are stored on the MedBike server) include:

- The session time and date
- The session mode as either clinical or single player
- The session duration
- The session biodata summary
    - The heart rate Min/Avg/Max values and % of blood oxygen saturation
    - The RPE peak value
    - The blood pressure (mmHg) at the beginning of the exercise, during the exercise, and after the exercise
- The bike session summary
    - Min/Avg/Max power and cadence
    - Total displacement performed during the exercise in the virtual world

- Full ECG data documentation:
    - A complete ECG recording of the session, viewable on a mm-calibrated grid;
    - Annotated ECG recording;
- Clinician session notes

2.3 Patient privacy and data integrity

MedBike system was designed to guarantee patient's privacy and data integrity. This is critical as MedBike runs on public networks. MedBike preserves patient's data

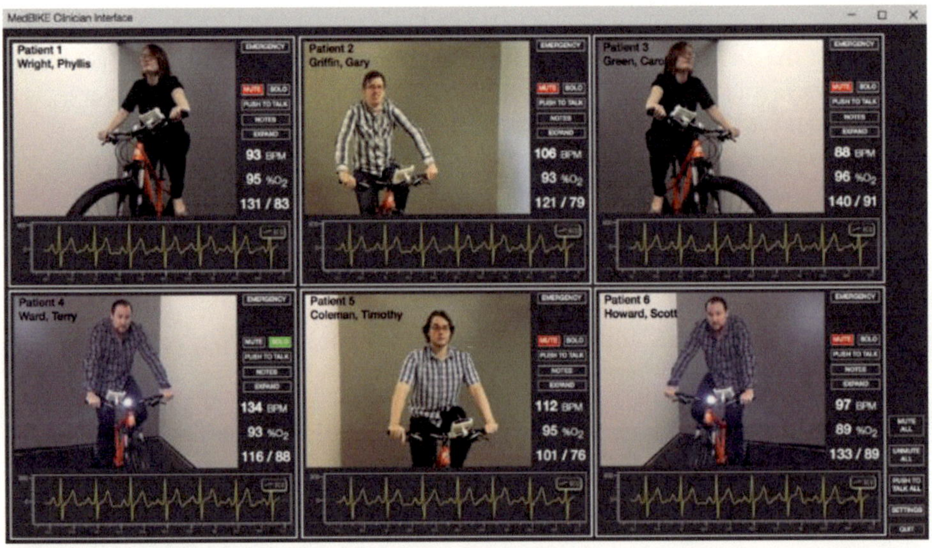

Figure 6.
Clinician's display showing six patients in a session.

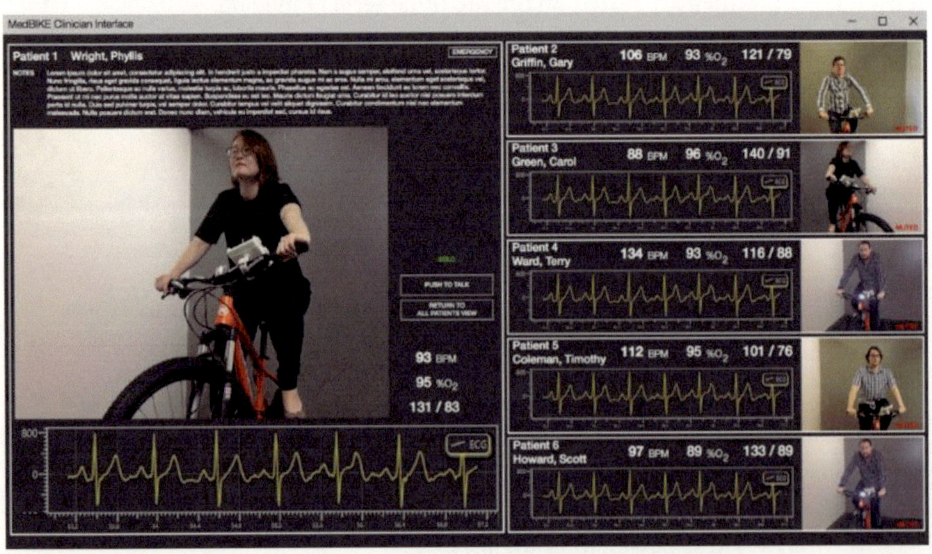

Figure 7.
Clinician's display focusing on one patient.

privacy in two ways (see **Figure 8**). MedBike data are transmitted to a cloud-based data server, located in a secure location near the hospital, using a HTTPS encryption scheme. Using this scheme, the clinician and patient can exchange a new encryption key every session. The communication between MedBike and the cloud-based data server is hidden to port scanning using a virtual peripheral network (VPN). Once the encrypted connections are established with each patient, the clinician can then monitor them in full confidence. Because the clinician operates the system from within the hospital intranet, it is also possible to access the patient medical records in full security. Access to the patient medical records is critical to the rehabilitation process as it will allow the clinician to define specific exercise programs for each patient based on their physical condition. To validate data integrity, during a session, the clinician can observe the values of the bio-sensors and determine if they are in acceptable ranges. In addition, transmission errors of the data sent from patient to clinician can be detected using the integrity mechanisms built into the AES-GCM cipher used for encryption. As for the data integrity uploaded to the cloud-based server the system rely on the inherent validation process of the HTTPS services.

2.4 MedBike bandwidth requirement

As part of our initial design, we had to guarantee that MedBike could operate on the average home networking environments (~5 Mbps). In MedBike most of this bandwidth is used by WebRTC at a video resolution of 640 × 480 pixels. Additional bandwidth is required to upload files to the cloud-based server every 2 min. The largest file is for the ECG data with a size of 500 kB per file (with an ECG sampling rate of 100 Hz). If one counts all data transfers, MedBike requires a total bandwidth of 2.5 Mbps up/down which is well in the range of home networking.

2.5 Virtual reality rendering using MedBike data

In this project, we have used Unity 3D version 5.3 game engine to display to the patient a virtual world composed of trees, terrains, roads, and avatars representing other patients. One can see in **Figure 5** a typical patient's display with the virtual world rendering and session information.

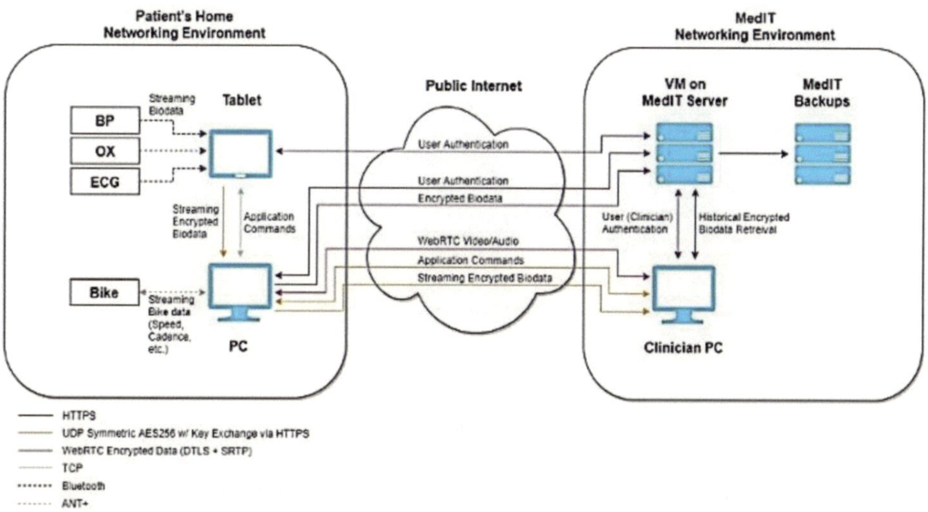

Figure 8.
MedBike secure networking.

To integrate the MedBike data (resistance, cadence, and steering) into the Unity 3D environment, we created new classes of objects that control the virtual camera in accordance to the avatar representing the patient.

Virtual Camera Update: By using bike speed and steering sensor measurements, one can change the new virtual camera position and direction to reflect the motion of the patient. The new position $\vec{p}(u(t+\Delta t), v(t+\Delta t))$ of the virtual camera is defined by:

$$\vec{p}(u(t+\Delta t), v(t+\Delta t)) = \vec{t}(u(t) + (c(t)\Delta t \cdot d_u(t)), v(t) + (c(t)\Delta t \cdot d_v(t)) + \vec{p}(u(t), v(t)) \quad (1)$$

where $\vec{p}(u(t),v(t))$ is the current position of the virtual camera relative to the digital terrain defined by a parametric surface $\vec{t}(u,v)$ where (u, v) are the parametric coordinates of the surface. The variables $c(t)$ is the bike speed as measured by the sensor and $(d_u(t), d_v(t))$ is the change in direction as measured by the rotary encoder. The rotary encoder has a resolution 1440 data points per revolution, which allows for an accuracy of 0.25 degrees. The rotary encoder is connected to a high-speed Phidgets encoder interface board connects directly to the PC via USB. A Phidgets API is used to read data from the encoder. The encoder is coupled to the steering column to detect rotation. One can see in **Figure 9** a close look at the rotary encoder setup.

Computing resistance: To compute the resistance that the KICKR must apply to the bicycle back wheel, a complex haptic rendering algorithm must be used (see **Figure 10**). The algorithm is initialized with a target power specified by the clinician, the minimum allowable resistance, the speed as measured by the KICKR, the current power produced by the patient, and the back wheel circumference. The resistance applied to the bicycle back wheel is continually adjusted to help the rider achieve a target power output. This allows workloads to be specified in Watts instead of arbitrary resistance values.

The resistance applied is calculated as follows. If linear speed is ≤ 0.025 m/s the resistance is held at the minimum allowed resistance. Otherwise, the target resistance value (R_{target}) is updated to the resistance value delayed by 1 second ($R_{delayed}$) plus or minus a small increment depending on the different between the power reported by the trainer and the target power output. The current resistance value applied by the bike trainer is then linearly interpolated toward the target resistance by 5%.

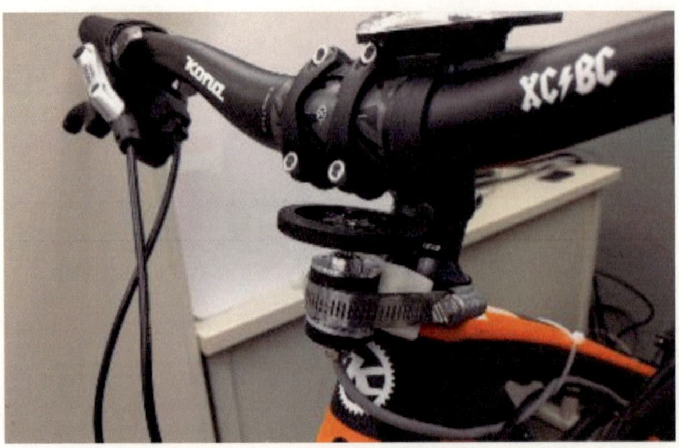

Figure 9.
Rotary encoder setup.

2.6 Multiplayers capability

In addition to the audio-visual connection (using WebRTC) between the clinician and each patient, each patient can see the avatars of the other patients using the

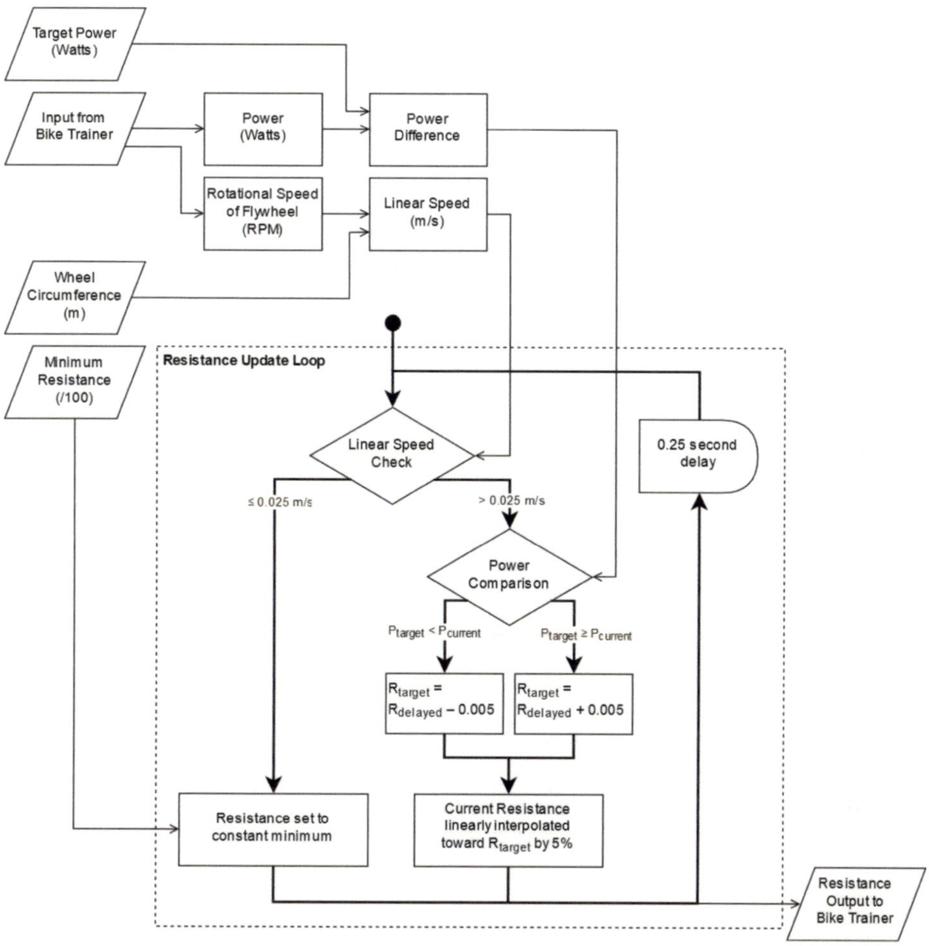

Figure 10.
MedBike resistance controller algorithm.

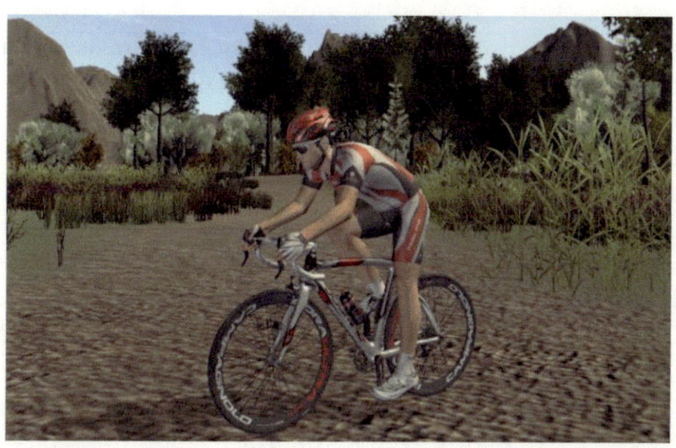

Figure 11.
Remote patient represented as an articulated avatar.

multiplayer capabilities of Unity 3D. At each patient's location, the avatars are fully animated and allow each patient to cycle and communicate with the other patients as a group. One can see at **Figure 11** a typical avatar representation. Each patient is personalized by changing the avatar's bike and cycling garment colors.

3. VR gamification to encourage adherence

Gamification has already been used in other telerehab programs for improving motor movement following surgical intervention [28, 29] and have shown to improve greatly adherence.

The first version of the VR simulation was built to represent a real-world outdoor biking experience. This virtual world consisted of beautiful trees, lakes, and mountains (see **Figure 5**) that the patient could explore at their own leisure alone or with another participant represented as a virtual avatar. No gaming aspect was added to this first version. Extremely positive feedback was received toward the experience, particularly being connected with a guiding clinician during weekly sessions. However, this VR world was limited in its ability to provide entertainment to the patient, an element we believe is truly important for establishing ongoing compliance to exercise CR programs. Two new VR worlds were developed to leverage the advantages of gamification.

Game for Pediatric Cardiac Patients: A VR world was developed for a pediatric cardiac rehabilitation program with a gaming environment specifically designed to engage child users into following a rehabilitation program (see **Figure 12**). The new game was designed for children with single heart ventricles who have undergone a corrective Fontan procedure and are severely deconditioned. Because of the high intensity interval training required for those patients, the game has two modes that alternate from a rest period to high-intensity exercise period. During the rest periods, the game requires that the patient explore the virtual world and collect strange roaming animals in order to acquire points. During the high intensity exercise periods, the patient must chase an animal into a wormhole by increasing their cadence to a specific level that if reached will eventually transport the user to a new world. The game for this project was created to integrate flawlessly into an exercise program designed specifically to train individuals with this condition. Furthermore, with the other inclusive features, such as remote monitoring (ECG and SpO_2), one can suggest the safety of higher exercise exertion in these children, which may convince parents to encourage more aggressive uptake of daily physical activity for their children. Exercise tolerance is strongly correlated with long term health outcomes; thus, individuals with significantly reduced capabilities such as Fontan patients, should be directed to improve their baseline exercise levels [30]. This project is of particular importance, as there is currently no cardiac rehabilitation standard protocol for pediatric patients, particular those with a history of a Fontan procedure. Thus, this project will assist in providing an evidence base for pediatric cardiac rehabilitation programs.

Virtual Spin-Class: With the great ability of Unity 3D to develop rapidly various game scenarios, a third application of MedBike was developed for encouraging exercise for mild cardiac disease and others who would benefit from exercise participation. Using the multiplayer capability of Unity 3D, a *spin-class* version of the system was developed. The game consists of numerous bikes (currently max six bikes) to be connected via the internet to a central cloud-based game engine that allows registered participants to chase moving targets, or each other, and to score points depending on their physical performance measured by wireless ECG sensors. Each participant is represented by an avatar (like **Figure 11**) that can be

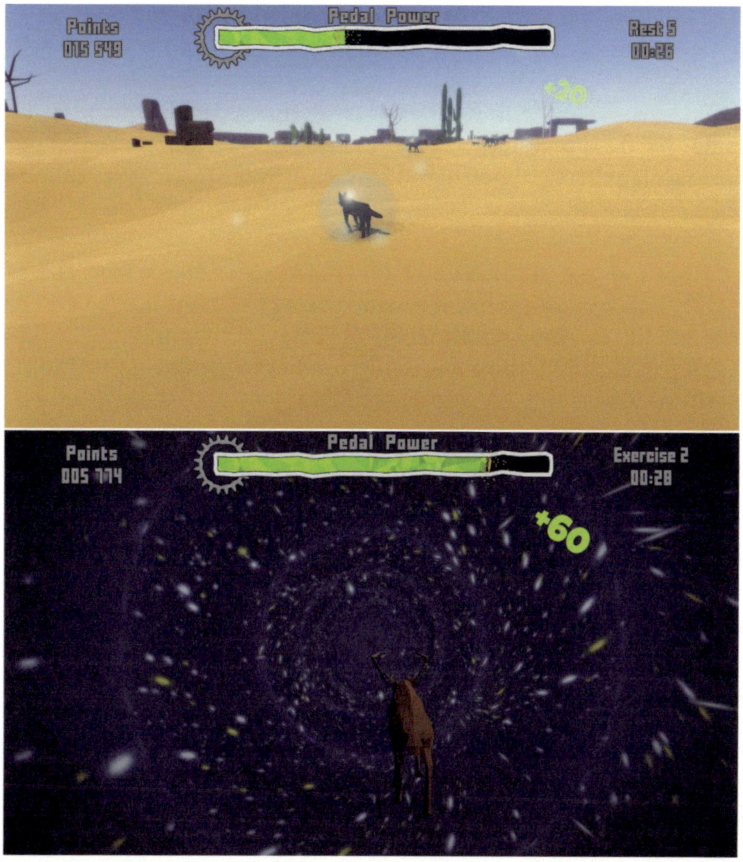

Figure 12.
Patient virtual reality experience for the pediatric rehabilitation game. The top image is during the rest phase and the bottom image is during the high intensity interval phase.

personalized at the beginning of the game. The virtual landscape is an island where participants must discover special targets that if collided with will cumulate points. The spin-class instructor can change the island level of difficulties by increasing the programmable bike resistance. The winner of the game will be the participant with the most points and with the best physical condition as measured by the sensors. In this version there is no clinician online. Instead, the sensor data is automatically analyzed by an advanced machine learning algorithm to determine exercise level performance and to detect from the ECG any abnormal condition that should be reported to the spin-class instructor and the participant. This version of MedBike will be deployed this summer at a local sports facility at the University of Alberta where it will be tested for usability and how it improves adherence to an exercise program.

4. Is MedBike effective for exercise-based cardiac rehabilitation?

4.1 A randomized pilot feasibility study

In 2017–2018, we conducted a small medical pilot project to assess:

1. The feasibility to perform home-based CR exercise using the MedBike system;

2. How MedBike can improve patient compliance to CR (frequency of exercise sessions and number of total hours spent exercising);

3. The effectiveness of MedBike at improving fitness levels (quantified using a standardized exercise tolerance test via a bicycle ergometer) and reduce cardiovascular risk (as determined by measuring BP, A1c, smoking status, and lipids).

We hypothesized that home-based CR using the MedBike system is feasible and will effectively improve program compliance using VR gamification and patient risk factor reduction by real-time monitoring. To prove this hypothesis 11 subjects (5 controls) were recruited into a feasibility randomized pilot control trial. Inclusion criteria was:

- Recent percutaneous cardiac intervention (PCI) or coronary artery bypass grafting (CABG);
- A left ventricular ejection fraction (LVEF) ≥45%;
- Internet connection (~5 mb/s download).

4.2 Feasibility study method

Each qualifying and consenting patient was enrolled in a standardized cardiac rehab program (based on the University of Alberta's Jim Pattison Centre for Heart Health protocol) consisting of 8 weeks of personalized exercise prescription. At the beginning of the study, patients were enrolled and randomized into the MedBike group, or standard of care group (control). Those randomized into the MedBike arm of the study were provided with the custom built MedBike VR exercise biking system with remote patient monitoring and clinical video conferencing; the standard of care group participated in a standard supervised exercise program carried out at the Jim Pattison Centre for Heart Health. In the MedBike group, the system was delivered to patient homes prior to the beginning of their first connected exercise session with the clinician. The control group received a standard exercise program which included one supervised in-hospital session per week, with a recommended additional four unsupervised exercise sessions, outside of the hospital. The additional four sessions were also recommended to the MedBike group with the option of using the MedBike system in the offline unsupervised mode (exercise data was still stored and sent to the MedBike server). Before beginning the exercise program, each patient was consulted with to design an exercise program that best allows for their clinical and physical development. Effort tolerance was largely based on an initial exercise tolerance test (ETT), which is used to direct the level to which the patient can begin their physical exercise regime. The ETT was also used to gauge exercise improvement during the study by performing a baseline and post-test at 8 weeks. During supervised sessions, the MedBike group used only the exercise bike. The control group were encouraged to only use cycling as their form of cardiorespiratory training during their hospital sessions, however, they were also given the option to perform, in addition, strength training and additional cardio exercises. This may have biased the comparison results of the ETT, but not the quantity or duration of total exercise performed over the 8 weeks. The MedBike platform was set up with the ability of the clinician to modify the exercise program and cycling resistance in real time, allowing for personalized program progression. Clinical communication was allowable through bi-directional video/audio feeds, whereby the clinical could communicate with one single patient individually or the group of patients collectively. The remote monitoring medical grade sensors of the system allowed for ongoing heart rhythm, blood pressure and oxygen saturation assessment; relevant data was selected from the session recordings and included in the custom report.

4.3 Feasibility study results

No difference in ETT improvement (1.69 vs. 1.57 min) was observed. On the other hand, MedBike patients exercise adherence and participation was higher:

- total number of hours exercised (318 vs. 239 hours);
- total number of exercise sessions (315 vs. 246);
- average sessions per subject (63 vs. 49.2);
- average number of sessions per week (7.88 vs. 6.15).

Since this was a small feasibility trial, it was not fully powered, nor was it reliable to calculate the statistical significance of our findings, but it did allow us to gain some preliminary information on efficacy trends. Our work suggested that:

- Using VR gamification MedBike system can increase individual exercise session adherence within the rehab program;
- The installation of MedBike in each home was relatively easy but better system diagnostic tools are needed to perform better on-site remote testing;
- We were able to demonstrate that MedBike can indeed be used by non-technical patients. Most patients had no problem starting the system and communicating with the clinician;
- Despite a few issues with unreliable home internet connections, the bandwidth of the average home internet services was enough to allow the clinician to perform rehabilitation sessions;
- The clinician interface and data display were sufficiently good to be useful during a session;
- Most of the patients enjoyed doing exercise using the virtual game.
- Many patients also greatly appreciated not having to go to the hospital to do the exercise program. They also appreciate not having to pay for parking and the system ability to integrate their rehab program into their lifestyle.

5. Conclusion

We presented in this paper the technical aspects and the measured performance of MedBike. Developing MedBike around Unity 3D has been an excellent design choice because of its flexibility and ease of programming new functions. In addition, Unity 3D is one of the video game industry standards and the development of additional games is relatively easy. During the pilot project in the patient's home, we were able to demonstrate that the system can work on a standard home internet connection. Before the medical pilot study, we performed numerous (40 persons) usability studies in our laboratory to optimize the interface design. Over 90% of the users of MedBike were very impressed by its performance and would certainly like to use it capabilities for their home exercise program if the system was not so expensive. The main reason for MedBike high-cost is because we use the KICKR from Wahoo and a relatively high-end mountain bike making the average price of the bike to be around $5 K CAN. By using low-cost stationary bikes ($265), a new low-cost ($300) resistance control system based on stepper motor controlling a simple bike, and a SONY Play station 4 ($350) instead of a graphic PC, we were able to design a low-cost system that will be below $1500.

The current version of MedBike has shown to be effective for delivering exercise programs to post procedural and event cardiac patients, saving time, encouraging adherence to the exercise program, and ensuring patient safety by direct clinician monitoring. We also believe that by adding a machine learning functionality that will analyze the MedBike biometric data in real-time to determine if the exercise level fits in the bounds of the prescribed exercise program safely, the system can be extensively used in sports facilities or at home to encourage higher activity levels in an older and detrained population.

Acknowledgements

This study has been funded by a grant from the University Hospital Foundation, University of Albert Hospital, and by an endowed research chair in healthcare solutions sponsored by CISCO Systems.

Author details

Pierre Boulanger[1*], William Mott[1], Stephanie Schaeffer[1], Peter W. Wood[2], Raj Padwal[2] and Paolo Raggi[2]

1 Department of Computing Science, University of Alberta, Canada

2 Department of Medicine, Faculty of Medicine and Dentistry, University of Alberta, Canada

*Address all correspondence to: pierreb@ualberta.ca

References

[1] Anderson L, Oldridge N, Thompson DR, Zwisler AD, Rees K, Martin N, et al. Exercise-based cardiac rehabilitation for coronary heart disease: Cochrane systematic review and meta-analysis. Journal of the American College of Cardiology. 2016;**67**:1-12

[2] Suaya JA, Shepard DS, Normand SL, Ades PA, Prottas J, Stason WB. Use of cardiac rehabilitation by medicare beneficiaries after myocardial infarction or coronary bypass surgery. Circulation. 2007;**116**:1653-1662

[3] Bjarnason-Wehrens B, McGee H, Zwisler AD, Piepoli MF, Benzer W, Schmid JP, et al. Cardiac rehabilitation in Europe: Results from the European cardiac rehabilitation inventory survey. European Journal of Cardiovascular Prevention and Rehabilitation. 2010;**17**:410-418

[4] Neubeck L, Freedman SB, Clark AM, Briffa T, Bauman A, Redfern J. Participating in cardiac rehabilitation: A systematic review and meta-synthesis of qualitative data. European Journal of Preventive Cardiology. 2012;**19**:494-503

[5] Doll JA, Hellkamp A, Ho PM, Kontos MC, Whooley MA, Peterson ED, et al. Participation in cardiac rehabilitation programs among older patients after acute myocardial infarction. JAMA Internal Medicine. 2015;**175**:1700-1702

[6] Jelinek MV, Thompson DR, Ski C, Bunker S, Vale MJ. 40 years of cardiac rehabilitation and secondary prevention in post-cardiac ischaemic patients. Are we still in the wilderness? International Journal of Cardiology. 2015;**179**:153-159

[7] Daly J, Sindone AP, Thompson DR, Hancock K, Chang E, Davidson P. Barriers to participation in and adherence to cardiac rehabilitation programs: A critical literature review. Progress in Cardiovascular Nursing. 2002;**17**:8-17

[8] Evenson KR, Fleury J. Barriers to outpatient cardiac rehabilitation participation and adherence. Journal of Cardiopulmonary Rehabilitation and Prevention. 2000;**20**:241-246

[9] Grace SL, Gravely-Witte S, Brual J, Monette G, Suskin N, Higginson L, et al. Contribution of patient and physician factors to cardiac rehabilitation enrollment: A prospective multilevel study. European Journal of Cardiovascular Prevention & Rehabilitation. 2008;**15**:548-556

[10] Tirrell BE, Hart LK. The relationship of health beliefs and knowledge to exercise compliance in patients after coronary bypass. Heart and Lung. 1980;**9**:487-493

[11] Dishman RK. Compliance/adherence in health-related exercise. Health Psychology. 1982;**1**:237-267

[12] Taylor RS, Dalal H, Jolly K, Moxham T, Zawada A. Home-based versus centre-based cardiac rehabilitation. Cochrane Database of Systematic Reviews. 2010;**1**:1-60

[13] Balady GJ, Ades PA, Bittner VA, Franklin BA, Gordon NF, Thomas RJ, et al. Referral, enrollment, and delivery of cardiac rehabilitation/secondary prevention programs at clinical Centers and beyond: A presidential advisory from the American Heart Association. Circulation. 2011;**124**:2951-2960

[14] Safiyari-Hafizi H, Taunton J, Ignaszewski A, Warburton DER. The health benefits of a 12-week home-based interval training cardiac rehabilitation program in patients with heart failure. The Canadian Journal of Cardiology. 2016;**32**(4):561-567

[15] Smolis-Bąk E, Dąbrowski R, Piotrowicz E, Chwyczko T, Dobraszkiewicz-Wasilewska B, Kowalik I, et al. Hospital-based and telemonitoring guided home-based training programs: Effects on exercise tolerance and quality of life in patients with heart failure (NYHA class III) and cardiac resynchronization therapy. A randomized, prospective observation. International Journal of Cardiology. 2015;**199**:442-447

[16] Rawstorn JC, Gant N, Direito A, Beckmann C, Maddison R. Telehealth exercise-based cardiac rehabilitation: A systematic review and meta-analysis. Heart. 2016

[17] Worringham C, Rojek A, Stewart I. Development and feasibility of a smartphone, ECG and GPS based system for remotely monitoring exercise in cardiac rehabilitation. PLoS ONE. 2011;**6**:e14669

[18] Lear SA, Singer J, Banner-Lukaris D, Horvat D, Park JE, Bates J, et al. Randomized trial of a virtual cardiac rehabilitation program delivered at a distance via the internet. Circulation Cardiovascular Quality and Outcomes. 2014;**7**:952-959

[19] Psotka J. Immersive training systems: Virtual reality and education and training. Instructional Science. 1995;**23**:405-431

[20] Annesi J, Mazas J. Effects of virtual reality-enhanced exercise equipment on adherence and exercise-induced feeling states. Perceptual and Motor Skills. 1997;**85**:835-844

[21] Laver K, George S, Thomas S, Deutsch JE, Crotty M. Cochrane review: Virtual reality for stroke rehabilitation. European Journal of Physical and Rehabilitation Medicine. 2012;**48**:523-530

[22] Laver K, George S, Thomas S, Deutsch JE, Crotty M. Virtual reality for stroke rehabilitation: An abridged version of a Cochrane review. European Journal of Physical and Rehabilitation Medicine. 2015;**51**:497-506

[23] Rhodesa R, Warburton D, Bredin S. Predicting the effect of interactive video bikes on exercise adherence: An efficacy trial. Psychology, Health & Medicine. 2009;**14**(6):631-640

[24] Mestre D, Maiano C, Dagonneau V, Mercier CS. Does virtual reality enhance exercise performance, enjoyment, and dissociation? An exploratory study on a stationary bike apparatus. Presence. 2011;**20**(1):1-14

[25] Fisher J, Thompson K, Nicoli L. Cardio-fitness station with virtual reality capability. US Patent, US 2007/0042868 A1; Feb. 22, 2007

[26] Nusbaum NH. Exercise bicycle virtual reality steering apparatus. US Patent, US 6,918,860 B1; Jul. 19, 2005

[27] Available from: http://www.widerun.com/

[28] Rybarczyk Y, Pérez Medina JL, Leconte L, Jimenes K, González M, Esparza D. Implementation and assessment of an intelligent motor tele-rehabilitation platform. Electronics. 2019;**8**(1):58. DOI: 10.3390/electronics8010058

[29] Rybarczyk Y, Kleine Deters J, Cointe C, Esparza D. Smart web-based platform to support physical rehabilitation. Sensors. 2018;**18**(5):1344. DOI: 10.3390/s18051344

[30] McCoy J, Bates M, Eggett C, Siervo M, Cassidy S, Newman J, et al. Pathophysiology of exercise intolerance in chronic diseases: The role of diminished cardiac performance in mitochondrial and heart failure patients. Open Heart. 2017;**4**(2)

Chapter 7

Restoring Independent Living after Disability Using a Wearable Device: A Synergistic Physio-Neuro Approach to Leverage Neuroplasticity

Subhasis Banerji, John Heng, Effie Chew, Christopher Wee Keong Kuah, Ling Zhao, Soh Yan Ming, Daphne Menezes and Ponvignesh Ponnusamy

Abstract

The number of people living with various grades of disability is now in excess of 1 billion. A significant portion of this population is dependent on caregivers and unable to access or afford therapy. This emerging healthcare challenge coincides with new knowledge about the self-learning, self-organizing, neuroplastic nature of the brain, offering hope to those trying to regain independence after disability. As conditions such as stroke and dementia begin to affect more and more people in the younger age groups, there is an urgent, global need for a connected rehabilitation solution that leverages the advantages of neuroplasticity to restore cognitive and physical function. This chapter explains a novel approach using a Synergistic Physio-Neuro learning model (SynPhNe learning model), which mimics how babies learn. This learning model has been embedded into a wearable, biofeedback device that can be used to restore function after stroke, injury, the degenerative effects of aging or a childhood learning disability. This chapter enumerates the clinical studies conducted with adult stroke patients in two scenarios—with therapist supervision and with lay person supervision. The results indicate that such a learning model is effective and promises to be an accessible and affordable solution for patients striving for independence.

Keywords: SynPhNe, stroke, rehabilitation, wearables, biofeedback, neuroplasticity, EEG, EMG, sensors

1. Introduction

In a systematic review of 151 studies, there was insufficient evidence that traditional neurological treatment methods were effective in improving muscle strength, synergies, muscle tone, dexterity, or ADLs after stroke [1]. Kollen et al. reviewed 735 available published (clinical) stroke rehabilitation trials [2]. They concluded that conventional treatment approaches induce improvements that are confined to impairment level only and do not generalize at a functional improvement level. In contrast, they stated that the treatment strategies that incorporate a strong emphasis on functional training may hold the key to optimal stroke rehabilitation and that appropriate intensity and task-specific exercise therapy are important components of such an approach. This was later reconfirmed to various degrees by others [3, 4].

Several commercially available devices have been built to deliver repetitive movements to an impaired human hand for stroke survivors to regain the use of the hand. However, the dysfunction of the natural afferent feedback pathways and proprioception hampers the sensory learning process of the patient and its conversion to execution of movement. This contributes to an inadequate restoration of functionality despite reducing impairment at a gross motor level [4, 5]. External manifestations of movement such as trajectory, force, acceleration, range of motion and the like are ultimately dependent on adequate, appropriate, and timely self-regulation of brain and muscle activity specific to various tasks. After an event such as stroke, various compensatory strategies come into play to execute the same movements, which, left unaddressed, become learned behavior. Re-engaging the human being's innate sensory learning mechanisms to regain the appropriate muscle and neural strategies is, therefore, a challenge and an unmet need. If high repetition-based rehabilitation is embarked upon without such re-learning, one runs the risk of post-trauma compensatory strategies being unknowingly reinforced in the brain, thus restoring movement and function in only a limited manner [6, 7].

1.1 Learning in a rehabilitation context

The body learns coordination for task performance by using all the lessons learnt from neuro-muscular, inter-limb, intra-limb, and eye-hand co-ordination [8, 9]. The specific strategies used are not only different from task to task for a person, but also differ for any one task between persons [10]. Initially, it was thought that the muscle synergies eliminated the redundant degrees of freedom by constraining the movements of certain joints or muscle [10]. But this does not work very well with the initial pathological constraints of an impaired arm. It has also been shown that constraining the movement of certain joints and muscles requires more energy and neural commands, and hence increases the number of neural signals required to perform the task [11]. However, some strategies are fundamental to all movement, such as maintaining an agonist-antagonist balance in the appropriate muscle groups, a moderation of effort to make repetitions possible during rehabilitation without being confounded by fatigue, and an active brain state which allows one to bring attention to the task at hand in a consistent manner. Facilitating such general strategies with technology rather than directly and artificially controlling individual, task-specific strategies is less complex, requires lower computational power and could facilitate a generalization of such useful strategies to other activities. This could in turn result in higher degrees of independence.

As an illustration, let us consider how humans learn handwriting. This is usually done by tracing over an existing alphabet or joining dots in the shape of an alphabet. Here, constraints are mind imposed based on visual cues while no constraints are placed physically on the hand. These mind-imposed constraints involve seeing a pattern and responding with a pencil, like a sort of static imitation. Everyone may choose a different strategy to impose these constraints, based on the kinematics of the more proximal joints and natural synergies of muscles proximal to the point where control is desired. This is like the uncontrolled manifold hypothesis for motor learning and involves a mechanism by which brain and body complement each other in real-time in managing elemental and contextual variables [12]. Hence, there does seem to be some convergence between motor learning theory and how developmental biology describes babies and infants learning in an associative, Hebbian manner using their sensory and motor faculties. The next question is whether such learning can be used as a pathway to undo the maladaptive, compensatory brain-muscle strategies that are common among chronic stroke patients with upper arm disability and help re-educate the adoption of appropriate strategies.

1.2 Self-regulation and its impact on learning and neuroplasticity

Stroke is an injury that affects not only body but also cognition and cardiovascular health, among others. Hence, it resembles a systemic injury or trauma even in mild to moderate cases. Healing of such systemic injuries has the final pathway of self-management or self-regulation [13, 14]. Self-regulation is ingrained by a biological, natural model of learning driven by the feedback and feedforward of information [13]. Self-regulation essentially requires a measure (absolute or relative), some facility to monitor changes in real-time, and some training to help develop the skill to modify the measure and move it in a desired direction [14, 15]. In the area of motor recovery, similar benefits of "self-control" have been demonstrated [16] but it is not very clear whether it can result in improvement in functional tasks.

Exercise is one way of providing an enriched motor environment. It facilitates plasticity in the brain and protects against the erosive effects, and this is one of the fundamental principles of early mobilization and continuing long term therapy. However, not all exercise regimens are adaptive, and some may even be maladaptive. In animal studies, the location and type of injury appear to dictate to some extent whether the intensity of motor rehabilitation training results in pro-plasticity, neutral or adverse contralesional hemisphere effects [17]. Additionally, the contralesional hemisphere appears to benefit from early, intense, motor enrichment while the perilesional area may be most helped by a gradual, modest increase in therapy. On another note, if the motivation to use the impaired limb after stroke is reduced due to ineptitude, pain or fatigue in that limb and there is a corresponding increased reliance on the other extremity, "learned non-use" of the impaired limb is the result [18].

While remarkable improvements in function have been reported when the non-impaired arm is constrained, as in constraint-induced therapy [19], excessively intense therapy can also lead to increased chances of secondary tissue loss due to reduction of brain derived neurotrophic factor (BDNF) expression in the brain during recovery [20]. Thus, while early onset of therapy using repetitive practice is vital to recovery, too much of it can exaggerate the extent of injury. This becomes even more significant because commonly used clinical assessment tests are not sensitive to small changes and do not allow the experimenter to distinguish between actual neurological recovery and behavioral compensation [21]. Just as neuroplasticity is a mechanism which can be leveraged to regain function, training of inappropriate, compensatory muscle and neural strategies, adopted unknowingly, can just as easily get ingrained in the brain and may take a long time to undo. The chances of this happening are heightened after stroke, when touch function, proprioception and cognition are adversely affected, and self-regulation ability is reduced due to the disruption of the natural feedback loops. Hence, apart from re-learning brain and muscle strategies, self-regulation of intensity in order to consistently keep compensation at bay and maintain beneficial strategies during training is another important component in this learning-led recovery model.

Like in the handwriting example given earlier, any learning model must satisfy the requirements of an experience derived from a sensory-rich system, as well as a motor system free of artificial constraints, which can adequately choose the synergy and/or strategy necessary to respond to this sensory system [22]. This is very similar to infants who learn in a non-instructional manner rich in sensory experience, using a feedforward-feedback sampling process [23]. Like in infants, the presence of such plasticity may provide an opportunity for functional recovery after stroke, if the most appropriate strategies are learnt and the maladaptive ones unlearnt [24].

2. The synergistic physio-neuro (SynPhNe) learning model

2.1 Learning in babies

There is now a growing understanding about how the body affects learning. The embodiment hypothesis proposes that sensorimotor activity of the person as it interacts with the environment is central to the development of intelligence [23]. In this field of study, the six principles of learning that babies instinctively follow can be summarized as under [23]:

1. Being multi-modal.
2. Being incremental.
3. Being physical.
4. Exploring.
5. Being social.
6. Learning a language (symbolic representation).

2.1.1 Being multi-modal

A multi-modal experience of the world is achieved in humans through the sensory system which is made up of a vast array of sensors to provide vision, audition, touch, smell, balance, and proprioception. Any single function can be accomplished by more than one signal configuration from the neurons and different neuron clusters need not be limited to a single function. This type of redundancy ensures continuity in function where parts of the network can learn from each other without an external teacher.

The second characteristic is the time-locked correlations between several simultaneous inputs, which are a powerful tool for representation, both singly and in combination with various events and objects in the environment [25]. In real-time these activities are mapped to each other to discover "higher order regularities," for example, using a combination of touch and vision to understand texture or transparency.

2.1.2 Being incremental

In non-incremental learning, the entire training set is usually fixed and then presented in entirety or randomly sampled. However, it seems that systematic changes in the input patterns and their overlapping occurrence in time play a large part in determining the development process. As a child grows, the vision starts to couple with the hearing and helps organize attention. In hearing-impaired babies, we see disorganized attention and a consequent slower learning (this is common in stroke cases, where patients experience sensory overload and cognitive deficiencies). Co-ordination is a form of mapping of multi-modal learning and the way they map changes over the development time, using either changing patterns or additional sensory inputs which the infants are now able to voluntarily provide themselves through physical exploration. Shifts in inputs thus result from the infant's own behavior. Using the body and moving from one place to another presents new spatial-temporal patterns and alters the infant's perception of "objects, space and self." Experimental studies show that one of the factors that strongly influence biological intelligence is "ordering the training experiences in the right way" [26].

2.1.3 Being physical

Experiments by Ballard et al. [27] and Baldwin [28] show that children off-load short term memory to the world by linking objects and events to locations, using attention to selectively point to the world. It is an easy way to build coherence in the cognitive system and to keep contents of different information clusters separate from each other.

2.1.4 Exploring

Initially the baby does not know what there is to learn. Babies can discover both the tasks to be learned and the solution to those tasks through exploration or non-goal directed action. One of the ways of exploration is spontaneous movement. As they contact objects in the environment, they progress from non-reaching to reaching. Thus, they seem to move from arousal to exploration to a selection of solutions from whatever space they can explore, which initially is limited. This type of learning is possible because of the multi-modal sensory system that builds maps from time-locked correlations starting with smaller spatial maps and expanding to larger ones.

2.1.5 Being social

In early interaction with mothers, infants learn from a pattern of activity that tightly couples vision, audition, and touch to behavior. Mother and infant imitate each other to reinforce this coupling. A mature social partner can also build a cognitive framework by weaving their own behavior around the child's natural activity patterns. This is done by automatically selecting those patterns which they consider meaningful and helpful for the baby. They also serve to direct attention to an object or event to strengthen the coupling. This is done in the spatial as well as temporal aspects. The baby frequently looks for physical and directional support to manage the risks around exploration, to rest when tired and to crystallize goals through such imitation and coupling.

2.1.6 Learning a language

Language can be a regularity that is a "shared communicative system." It is also a symbol system where the relation between the symbol and events in the world are mainly arbitrary, e.g., there is no relation between the word "dog" and what it represents, by knowing the word we cannot know the animal. DeLoache [29] demonstrated the way children use scale models and pictures as symbols which are not too life-like. Children first learn subtle regularities from the words they absorb, and slowly it creates in them the ability to learn a word in one trial and do higher-order generalization. Efficient learning through a form of language thus itself becomes learned behavior.

While new born babies have non-goal directed exploratory behavior, they soon graduate into a more goal-directed behavior. These goals are a result of their decision-making process which takes inputs from their emotions, knowledge, intelligence, and social partners (in this case maybe parents or elder siblings). The mature partner moderates the child's emotions and value system and therefore, his or her early decisions during the learning process. This may be done through instruction, dialogue, feedback, and body language.

When this is considered in the context of a stroke patient, the goals he or she sets for recovery would be influenced by the same factors and more so with increasing disability and physical and emotional dependence. If we break down the learning process into its two broad components, exploratory and goal-directed, then one can line up the two components as an illustration shown in **Figure 1**. The patient formulates a goal (as in recovery of a specific function such as eating) and can begin exploratory learning in that specific context. However, there may exist cognitive as well as physical and social constraints due to post-stroke disability. If a technology could augment these aspects so that constraints are reduced through an appropriately designed user interface, it may facilitate such a patient re-booting how he learnt as a baby.

The goal dictates the quality, direction, and extent of the exploration. In stroke patients, the immediate and longer-term goals that the patient sets for himself/herself could significantly affect extent and speed of recovery [30]. Behavior generation is built around a distributed network of responses such as approach, play, avoidance of obstacles and attention requisition, all of which may be affected adversely after stroke. Behaviors may excite or inhibit each other, where non-conflicting behaviors fire motor commands with the brain and muscle complementing each other in real-time.

2.2 Integrating learning into functional recovery

In a learning environment which requires multiple repetitions, not all of which are identical, as in re-learning a skill, **Figure 1** forms the basic element of the learning iterations. Several iterations will be required as part of the exploratory strategy over time, which may be represented by a cyclic model as shown in **Figure 2**. In this figure, the feedback and feedforward loops drive subsequent iterations, which may be similar or dissimilar. Goals and decisions, as a feedforward, drive multi-modal exploration. Incremental changes or achievements seen at brain and body levels through measurable and quantifiable feedback drive modifications in belief systems, thus impacting goals and decisions for further learning.

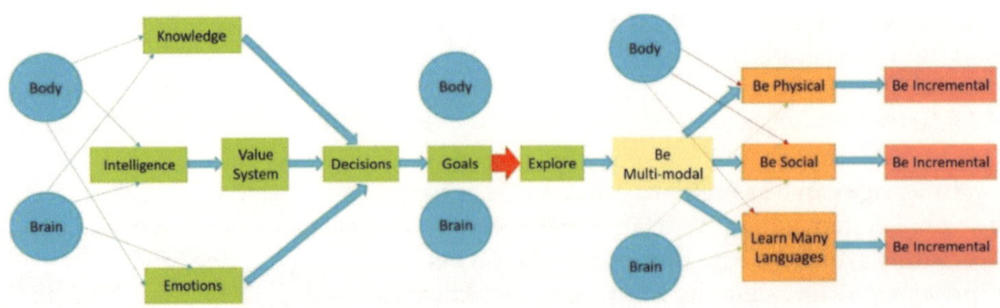

Figure 1.
A composite learning behavior using the mind and physical body in a multi-modal fashion for goal-oriented exploration.

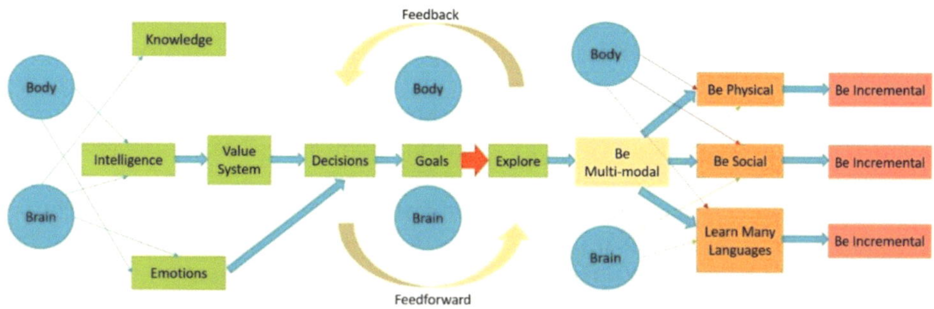

Figure 2.
The proposed natural learning model using iterative, incremental changes.

However, such faculties of learning available to a normal person may or may not be available to a stroke patient. A typical stroke model adapted from Ito et al. [31] of how stroke affects the human system resulting in motor function impairment is shown in **Figure 3** with an augmentation of such impaired feedforward and feedback superimposed. In this figure, the pathways for motor commands from motor cortex and proprioceptive feedback from the musculoskeletal system are disrupted and hence, some alternate pathway is recommended shown by the "motor intention" and "motor actuation" blocks. This is a popular model implemented by the rehabilitation robotics community and those adopting the stimulation approach. Motor intention is usually sensed by a brain-computer interface or artificially induced by stimulation methods such as transcranial magnetic stimulation. Motor actuation is achieved by either electrical stimulation or mechanically driven robotic movement. Intention and actuation are bridged typically by some adaptive algorithm which may be based on feature extraction, a control strategy, and a feedback

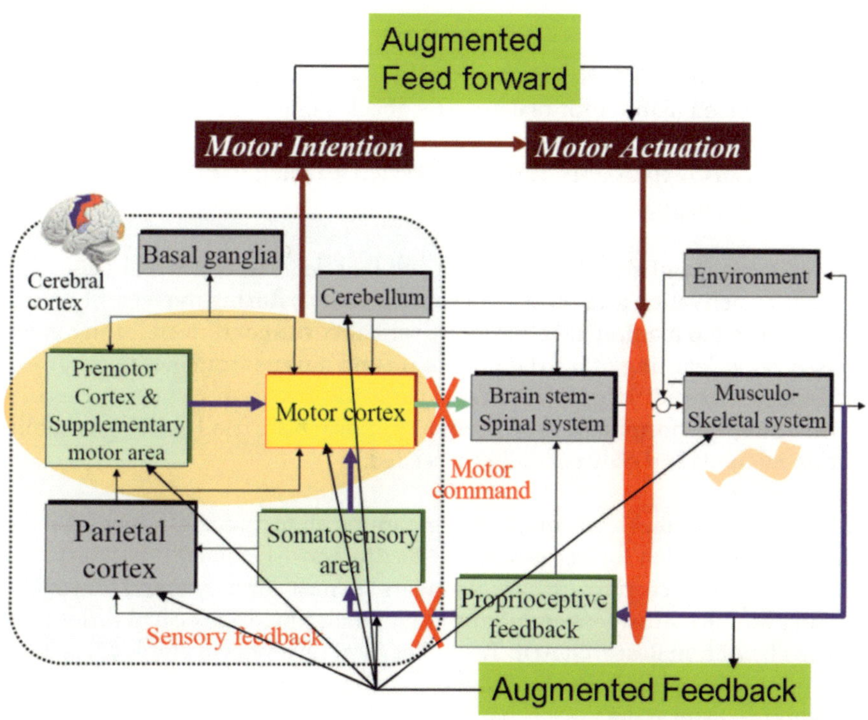

Figure 3.
The self-regulated model of recovery of motor impairment after stroke adapted from Ito et al. [31].

loop. Current technology, however, is not able to address the complex issue of hand function, which involves overlapping neuro-physio strategies and multiple degrees of freedom. At most, simple movements may be possible [32] which has been shown to not adequately impact function for the highly heterogeneous stroke affected population. Gross movements can be expected to improve with very high number of repetitions, thus enabling the brain to rewire itself in a limited way. However, there is poor evidence that such gross movement practice translates significantly into function. Therefore, the modification to the above model is proposed, incorporating the feedforward and feedback elements modeled in **Figure 2** as a form of augmentation to help overcome the deficits through the learning route.

The augmented feedback may be delivered visually via a muscle-brain-computer interface. The feedforward in the form of appropriate audio-visual inputs, which lead the human to attempt a series of desired actions through imitation, is known to facilitate recovery [33]. Moreover, there is evidence of perception transferring to action and more importantly, from action to perception [34]. The augmented feedback is expected to drive motor intention and exploration while the feedforward is expected to prime the brain for motor actuation and goal directed learning through imitation. From a functional improvement perspective, the augmented feedback may be customized for a person using time-locked parameters as follows:

1. EMG agonist-antagonist balance (muscle strategy).

2. EEG relaxation and attention states (brain strategy).

The brain and the body are inseparably linked, and both contribute significantly for neuroplasticity to occur and health parameters to improve [35]. Based on this understanding of how human learning may be applied practically in the context of post-stroke rehabilitation, this study was conceived with the following assumptions:

1. When EEG and EMG signals during activity are brought together in a time-synchronized manner for real-time feedback along with an audio-visual feedforward for imitation, it provides an opportunity for the patient to work with sensory, exploratory and goal-directed learning toward functional rehabilitation goals.

2. Displaying quantified, relative brain and muscle feedback in real-time while training activation and relaxation simultaneously during movement or while attempting to manipulate objects, will enhance the conditions for incremental associative learning of overlapping brain and muscle strategies to occur [36]. Under such conditions, subjects may potentially achieve systemic gains in functional performance, even though they may have tried existing rehabilitation methods and only partially succeeded.

This paper describes a bio-mechatronics approach to understanding where re-learning is misled or failing and uses a "feedforward-feedback" modality to help chronic stroke subjects train gross movements (as measured by Fugyl Meyer Upper Extremity Motor Assessment scale) and functional, timed-task capabilities (as measured by Action Research Arm Test). The SynPhNe system employs learning and training principles similar to that which babies seem to use in the design of its user interface, to leverage the mechanism of "self-regulation" or "self-correction." The study explores to what extent such real-time "self-correction" alone, in the absence of any form of external stimulation or robotic assistance, impacts the recovery of functional ability in the stroke impaired, as a prelude to building a safe, effective, easy-to-use technology which would be useful for patients to augment therapy hours at home.

3. Methods

3.1 Technology description

3.1.1 Design principles for SynPhNe system

At the time of development, motor theory, learning principles and stroke rehabilitation challenges listed in Section 1 suggested that the SynPhNe rehabilitation platform should facilitate such learning keeping in mind the constraints faced by stroke patients.

- EEG and EMG biofeedback with video-based feed-forward provided the multi-modal environment.

- Incremental learning—use of biofeedback to highlight small changes in the muscle and the brain signals with their transitions and associating this with the gross movements and tasks performed with various degrees of success.

- Exploratory learning, using the hand for real world tasks perceived as important but difficult (for example, use of chopsticks), as well as understanding how to achieve various relaxation and attention states while in dynamic movement using the feedforward-feedback modality.

- Simulation of a "mature social partner" or instructor, perhaps in the form of an instructor led video which a patient could watch and follow and the smiley icon which indicates the successful management of the desired brain state while executing physical tasks.

- Teaching a new, universal language, i.e., making the subject aware of how to interpret and self-regulate muscle and brain activity at a signal level.

- Following the cyclic learning process shown in **Figure 2**, as a sensory-led, intuitive, self-sustaining, and reinforcing cycle.

3.1.2 System description

The wearable data capture unit (WDCU) acquires data from eight channels of EMG through an arm gear and eight channels of EEG data through a head gear and transmits the data simultaneously to the PC using a USB cable (**Figure 4**). The design of this arm gear has been previously reported in a separate paper by the authors along with design and testing of the amplification circuit [37]. The software running on the PC processes these signals from 16 channels and combines them in a time locked manner for presentation on the screen as real-time feedback showing muscle over-activation and under-activation as cartoon characters (EMG signal as agonist-antagonist koala bears climbing up or down a tree, EEG signal as a smiley face). While EMG signals are used as feedback by squaring and averaging the amplitude within a running window updated every 10 milliseconds, the EEG signals were converted to frequency band using a Fast Fourier Transform and the alpha

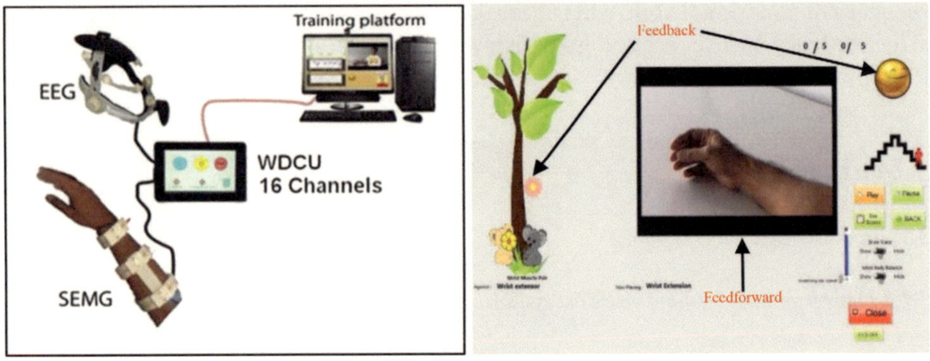

Figure 4.
SynPhNe learning model platform and user-interface.

band power (8–13 Hz) was used to represent a relaxed state, updated every 10 s as a proportion to total power in the 1–35 Hz frequency band. While EMG was sampled at 1000 samples/sec, EEG was sampled at 256 samples/s.

The goal of both the feedforward and feedback is to successfully attempt a movement or physical task while maintaining a relaxed brain-muscle state pre- and post-action comparable to resting state. If effort results in a deviation from resting state, return to resting state post-effort should be immediate. Brain and muscle influence each other too. Losing attention partially or fully may result in loss of ability to imitate the feedforward video and respond to feedback. Incremental changes in self-regulation are presented visually in the real-time user interface, which then provides an impetus for the patient to self-regulate further.

Figure 4 depicts the user interface on the computer screen. The subject observes the video as the feedforward in order to imitate it with the same speed. The koala bears, and tree serve as agonist and antagonist muscle EMG feedback during such imitation. The subject attempts to activate the appropriate muscle to raise the brown bear (agonist) to the top of the tree while keeping the gray bear (antagonist) as steady and close to the bottom of the tree as possible. The yellow smiley face represents EEG frequency band feedback as a measure of a relaxed brain state which needs to be maintained as best as possible while imitating the video-based physical movement or task.

In both the clinical studies, the subject tried to imitate an exercise and task practice video sequence running on the computer screen, while attempting to correct maladaptive over-activation and under-activation in opposing muscle pairs displayed on the same screen. Using a slower speed of execution than normal allowed proximal joints of the upper limb to stabilize and reduce temporal demands on the subject [38]. The slow-paced video sequences allowed time to train relaxation between repetitions. Also, the need to achieve a relaxation goal immediately after activation encouraged the subjects not to over-activate the muscles and to moderate their effort. This strategy was found to delay the onset of high dynamic muscle tone and allow for better repetition-based performance based on greater number of successful relaxations. When subjects experienced difficulties in being able to relax their muscles, they intuitively made postural corrections to let go and relax deeper before the next muscle activation. EMG thresholds displayed on the software gave them a clear indication on activation and relaxation targets appropriate for training, which were based on previously calibrated maximum voluntary contraction (targets were up to 40% of maximum) and resting state EMG respectively, for various muscle groups. In this paper, analysis of only the EMG peaks data as seen during activity and immediately post activity repetition is highlighted. The EEG and other metrics will be reported separately in subsequent papers since the primary objective of this paper is to highlight the thinking behind the user-interface design and the pre and post clinical outcomes.

3.2 Study methodology

In Trial 1, 15 adult chronic stroke subjects with a hemiplegic hand (31–69 years; 4 females, 11 males) were recruited for the study (**Table 1**). In Trial 2, 10 adult

Subject code	Age	Gender	Months poststroke	Nature of stroke
Demographics of subjects in Trial 1				
RH001	57	Female	22	Hemorrhage
RH002	44	Male	21	Infarct
RH003	54	Male	12	Infarct
RH004	61	Male	25	Infarct
RH005	69	Male	21	Infarct
RH006	38	Male	18	Hemorrhage
RH007	48	Male	18	Hemorrhage
LH001	31	Female	32	Infarct
LH002	53	Female	18	Hemorrhage
LH003	59	Female	37	Infarct
LH004	62	Male	8	Infarct
LH005	57	Male	10	Hemorrhage
LH007	65	Male	45	Hemorrhage
LH008	62	Male	15	Hemorrhage
Mean	54.3		21.6	
Std. dev.	10.3		10.0	
Demographic details of subjects in Trial 2				
NRH001	69	Male	21	Infarct
NRH002	60	Male	28	Infarct
NRH003	57	Female	23	Hemorrhage
NRH004	59	Male	7	Infarct
NRH005	65	Male	7	Infarct
NRH006	46	Male	60	Hemorrhage
NRH007	67	Male	49	Infarct
NLH001	61	Male	21	Infarct
NLH002	45	Male	49	Infarct
NLH003	62	Male	69	Infarct
Mean	60.0		32.3	
Std. dev	7.6		20.7	

Table 1.
Demographic of recruited subjects.

chronic stroke subjects with a hemiplegic hand (45–69 years; 1 female, 9 males) were recruited for the study (**Table 1**).

Both left and right limb impaired subjects were included for a better patient representation with at least 6 months post a first clinical stroke. Only paralysis with M.R.C. grade between 1 and 3 at elbow and digits was considered for inclusion. Passive, pain-free range of motion was at least 50% in all below elbow joints. No exclusion was made based on type of stroke and the group included those with ataxia and tactile sensory loss.

The experiments had only treatment group whose members had plateaued (those who had completed the rehabilitation program recommended by the hospital) in functional recovery and were ready to discontinue any other form of regular or alternative therapy during the study.

In Trial 1, the subjects were randomized between two clinical therapists, where either of them could conduct any session for any subject (as is common in a typical clinical setting). In Trial 2, to simulate a home-based, non-clinical environment, the therapy was not conducted in a standard hospital therapy/rehabilitation ward but rather in a normal spare room with a table and a chair. A research associate with a non-therapy background was trained to operate the SynPhNe system to deliver the sessions every day.

Each subject completed a 4-week, 3 sessions/week protocol using the automated SynPhNe device which delivers the learning modality. Each session lasted for 50–75 min including the setup time. In Trial 1, the EEG signals were captured during three sessions to track changes, i.e., in the beginning, midway and end of the study whereas in Trial 2, the EEG signals were captured in all 12 sessions, with the smiley face retained as a form of feedback on relaxed brain state represented by the relative alpha-band power as calibrated at rest. This brain-based feedback was introduced after it was observed that a significant component of therapist supervision in Trial 1 consisted of repeatedly nudging the subjects' attention back to task.

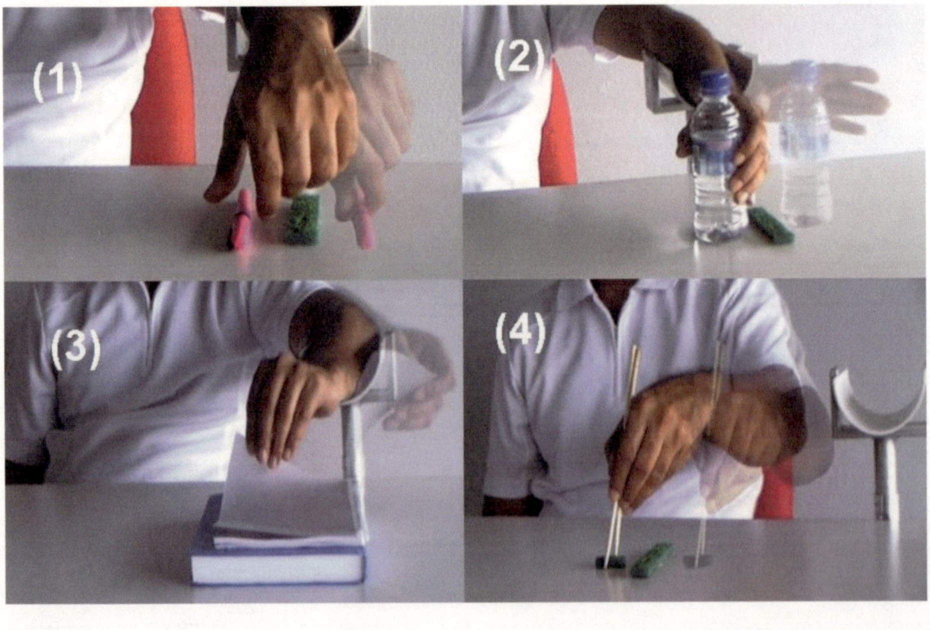

Figure 5.
Task practice (1) picking up a pen, (2) grasping a bottle, (3) flipping a page, (4) using a pair of chopsticks (pictures extracted from the instructional video created for the experiment).

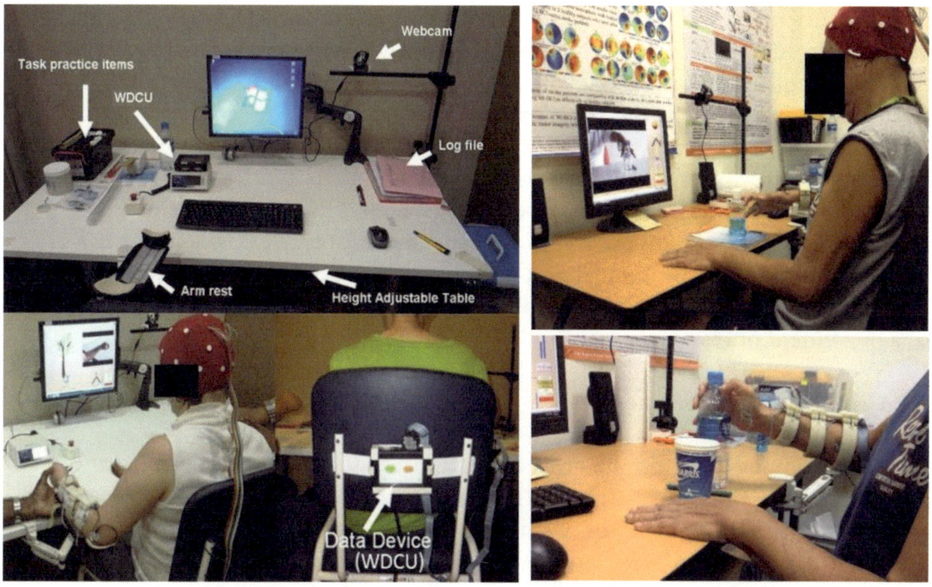

(A) (B)

Figure 6.
Clinical trial setup in (A) Trial 1 (therapy ward) and (B) Trial 2 (outside therapy ward).

Imitating the video, subjects performed four basic hand movements—wrist extension and flexion, finger extension and flexion, pronation and supination, and open grasp. This was followed by four everyday tasks—picking up a pen, flipping a page, grasping a bottle and use of chopsticks (**Figure 5**).

These four tasks were chosen to represent a two-finger pinch with pronation, a cylindrical grasp, a key pinch with pronation and supination and a five-finger pinch which demands attention. Each exercise was repeated five times in the first three sessions and 10 times in the subsequent sessions while attempting to maintain a pre-calibrated agonist-antagonist balance using the biofeedback. In Trial 1, some of the more severely affected subjects (n = 7) were provided the facility for an automated triggering of electrical stimulation on extensor muscles for some or all sessions if the subject achieved an agonist EMG threshold while maintaining a relaxed antagonist [39]. In Trial 2, we did not use any FES as Trial 1 indicated that FES induced exaggerated, instantaneous antagonist-side reactions, which our protocol was, in fact, trying to minimize.

Pre-, mid-, and post-outcomes were measured using standard clinical scales [Fugl Meyer Upper Extremity Motor assessment (FMA) and Action Research Arm Test (ARAT)] to assess both gross and fine movements [40]. They were also randomized for assessment between two other therapists who were blinded to the study protocol. All subjects provided a signed written consent. Ethics approval was obtained from the Institutional Review Board of National Healthcare Group, Singapore. The set-up for the two experiments is shown in **Figure 6**.

4. Results and discussions

4.1 Association of muscle contraction to relaxation

On comparing the muscle activation and relaxation scores across all subjects in Trial 1 (168 sessions) and Trial 2 (total 120 sessions), it was seen that successful performance of higher repetitions of muscle contractions above an EMG threshold was associated with the ability to volitionally relax those muscles below an EMG threshold immediately after contraction (Trial 1: Pearson's coefficient = 0.78, CI = 99%; Trial 2: Pearson's coefficient = 0.74, CI = 99%).

Subjects who were unable to relax, volitionally, in a consistent manner had difficulties in performing simple actions such as extensions and flexions repeatedly as well as tasks. The antagonist was observed to be relatively stronger (the gray koala bear climbed higher up on the tree) in most subjects at week 0, whenever the subjects tried to activate the agonist and raise the golden koala bear up the tree. These subjects also demonstrated an inability to relax a muscle immediately on completion of a movement or task.

4.2 Clinical scale outcomes

The outcomes based on the FMA and ARAT clinical scales for both the trials are summarized in **Table 2**. Subjects have been categorized into mildly- (55–57), moderately- (32–54) and severely-impaired (≤31) based on their FMA scores at week 0. Subject LH006 encountered a personal accident at home resulting in a head injury during the study and was discontinued from the trial.

The scores for both the assessment scales were reduced to a common denominator by normalizing assessment scores against full scores of the respective scale. For FMA and ARAT, the full scores are 66 and 57 respectively.

Based on the nominalized scores, the percentage improvement in both the functional scales for the subjects in Trial 1 and Trial 2 can be summarized as shown in **Table 3**. Since these improvements are based on initial measurements of level of impairment (week 0), they capture both clinical and sub-clinical performance changes or incremental improvements or decline achieved by the subjects. The estimated minimum clinically important difference (MCID) of the upper limb FMA scores ranges from 4.25 to 7.25 points depending on the different facets of upper limb movement (overall upper limb function MCID is 5.25) while the MCID values for the ARAT were 5.7 points for chronic stroke patients [41, 42]. In Trial 1, there were two subjects who achieved MCIDs in FMA; RH003 (8 points) and RH007 (9 points) and four subjects who achieved MCIDs in ARAT; RH005 (7 points), LH005 (7 points), LH007 (12 points), LH003 (6 points). In Trial 2, subjects NRH006 (13 points), NLH003 (6 points), NRH001 (7 points) and NRH003 (6 points) achieved MCIDs in ARAT. These MCIDs were achieved with only 5–10 repetitions per exercise per session, which is about 10–30% of the number of exercise repetitions recommended per session in standard care.

Training in self-regulation of antagonist muscle relaxation during movement using the SynPhNe system contributed to positive pre-post changes in FMA (Trial 1: Mean = 6.855%, SD = 7.85; Trial 2: Mean = 5.05%, SD = 6.00) and ARAT (Trial 1: Mean = 25.84%, SD = 49.86; Trial 2: Mean = 30.17%, SD = 21.20).

4.3 Discussions

Results from the two separate trials are presented to illustrate the degree of consistency in two different patient samples. The inclusion and exclusion criteria in both studies were similar. However, in Trial 1 therapists fully supervised the therapy sessions while in Trial 2 non-therapists conducted the sessions. In both studies, a separate team of blinded therapists performed the pre- and post-assessments. Neither study reported any adverse events.

Impairment level	Subject code	Fugl Meyer (FMA)		Action research arm test (ARAT)	
		W0	W4	W0	W4
Clinical outcomes in Trial 1					
Mild	RH001	58	60	53	57
Moderate	RH003	36	44	9	11
	RH005	45	46	20	27
	RH007	50	59	45	49
	LH001	35	33	5	5
	LH002	44	45	25	28
	LH004	45	44	21	21
	LH005	52	56	32	39
	LH007	50	52	32	44
	LH008	43	47	32	32
Severe	RH002	16	19	6	7
	RH004	27	27	5	5
	RH006	29	31	17	17
	LH003	22	24	3	9
Mean		39.43	41.93	21.79	25.07
Std. dev		11.86	12.67	15.10	16.64
Clinical outcomes in Trial 2					
Moderate	NRH006	54	56	38	51
	NLH003	43	42	17	23
	NLH002	38	41	25	28
	NRH001	38	40	18	25
	NRH007	37	39	21	26
	NRH004	37	39	27	31
	NRH003	32	33	7	13
Severe	NRH005	31	30	9	10
	NRH002	20	24	8	9
	NLH001	19	20	3	4
Mean		34.90	36.40	17.30	22.00
Std. dev		9.78	9.69	10.31	13.05

Table 2.
FMA and ARAT clinical scores at week 0 (W0) and week 4 (W4).

Figure 7 supported the research group's direction that both activation and relaxation must be trained specifically, as opposed to a pre-occupation with repeated muscle activation alone as is common in rehabilitation [43].

Both the studies reported a larger increase in ARAT scores as compared to FMA scores. This increase in ARAT was not necessarily linked to those who had high FMA scores at week 0. This suggests that functional task performance and object manipulation ability may improve even though reduction of impairment at a gross

Subject code	Fugl Meyer (FMA)	Action research arm test (ARAT)
Percentage improvement in Trial 1		
RH001	3.45	7.55
RH002	18.75	16.67
RH003	22.22	22.22
RH004	0.00	0.00
RH005	2.22	35.00
RH006	6.90	0.00
RH007	18.00	8.89
LH001	−5.71	0.00
LH002	2.27	12.00
LH003	9.09	200.00
LH004	−2.22	0.00
LH005	7.69	21.88
LH007	4.00	37.50
LH008	9.30	0.00
Mean	6.85	25.84
Std. dev	7.85	49.87
Percentage improvement in Trial 2		
NRH001	5.26	38.89
NRH002	20	12.5
NRH003	3.13	85.71
NRH004	5.41	14.81
NRH005	−3.23	11.11
NRH006	3.7	34.21
NRH007	5.41	23.81
NLH001	5.26	33.33
NLH002	7.89	12
NLH003	−2.33	35.29
Mean	5.05	30.17
Std. dev	5.72	20.22

Table 3.
Percentage improvement post-therapy (week 4) with respect to pre-therapy.

level is proportionately lower. Subjects who achieved MCIDs did so mostly in ARAT and not FMA, which is somewhat counter-intuitive. This may be because several functional tasks do not demand a full range of motion, e.g., Eating with chopsticks or Picking up a small object like a pen with a two-finger pinch. In the experience of the study team, it was noted that subjects were more motivated attempting to do actual functional tasks such as opening a book and manipulating chopsticks as compared to standard joint extension/flexion exercises that were repetitive and not directly linked to a perceived functional outcome. It may be noted that each exercise

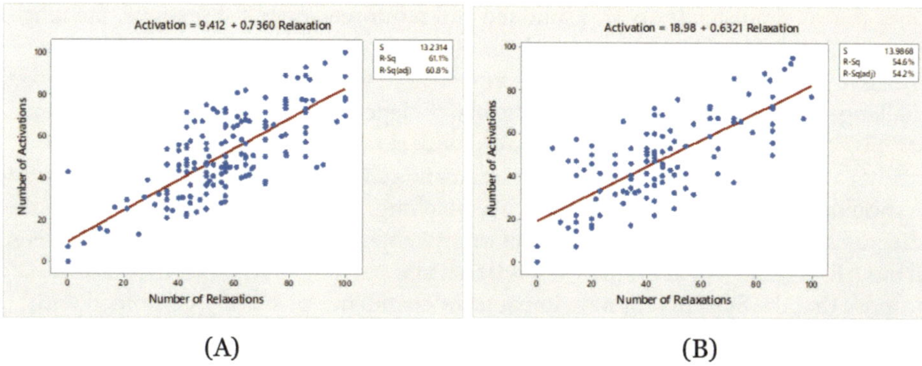

Figure 7.
Muscle activation is associated with relaxation during repetitive practice in (A) Trial 1 (B) Trial 2.

and activity was repeated only 5–10 times per session to produce the outcomes reported, which was about a fifth of the number usually recommended in rehabilitation settings, and about a tenth or less of that in high repetition therapy. This was done to ensure that compensatory strategies did not set in due to fatigue, boredom, or distraction. The results raise some questions about initial functional results being dependent on high repetitions and are, in fact, reminiscent about how babies learn with few, non-similar repetitions [29]. Since both studies exclusively recruited patients who were both chronic and plateaued, the chances of spontaneous recovery were minimized, although cannot be ruled out. The authors are of the opinion that restoration of function resembling spontaneous recovery may, in fact, be facilitated in the chronic phase of therapy by the re-learning of such brain and muscle strategies as described in these experiments, enhancement of relaxation and attention and the progressive reduction of compensation.

The gold standard for restoration of function and independence is still conventional, manual therapy. Kollen et al. reviewed more than 700 published studies and concluded that conventional robotic or stimulation treatment approaches induce improvements that are confined to impairment level only and do not generalize to functional improvement [2]. They stated that treatment strategies that incorporate a strong emphasis on functional training and task-specific therapy may hold the key to optimal stroke therapy. A search of systematic reviews in the Cochrane and other databases on well-known approaches such as electro-mechanical and robot-assisted arm training, electro-stimulation and EMG triggered neuromuscular stimulation of wrist and fingers showed that only electro-stimulation held certain advantages over conventional, manual therapy when comparing outcomes for motor ability [44–48]. However, conventional therapy continues to be superior in improving the complete spectrum ranging from gross motor, fine motor, strength, dexterity and ability to manipulate objects and perform timed tasks. Hence, the authors of this paper carried out a follow-up study with 30 subjects, comparing a group undergoing SynPhNe training to a group receiving standard care, which was a mix of conventional physiotherapy, physical therapy, occupational therapy and neuro therapy. Since the goal is to develop a system which can augment therapy effectively at home, the study was designed to prove that SynPhNe treatment was comparable to standard care. The results of this study have been published previously [49]. The conclusion was that SynPhNe training was comparable to standard care as seen in the FMA and ARAT scales.

The EMG data demonstrated that the stroke subjects had hitherto unknown antagonist over-activation in wrist and finger movements, which were moderated and subdued by starting the exercises with a reduced range of motion and reduced speed.

Once the antagonist activity was subdued and reinforced over 2–4 sessions, the range of motion and speed was progressively increased in subsequent sessions. This was effective particularly in wrist and finger extension, which is known to be a significant challenge for most stroke patients. Control deficiencies in approach, sequential steps and object release were similarly improved with slower execution speeds that were meant to effect better proximal stabilization and reduced compensation as often seen in shoulder elevation and abduction while reaching, pronating, and grasping with the affected arm. Since the most significant improvements in percentage terms were seen in the ARAT scale which evaluates functional and participation tasks, the authors propose that the SynPhNe system impacts independence positively, combined with enhanced self-regulation and the self-use of technology.

All subjects tolerated the multi-modal feedback well and did not report feeling overwhelmed by the user interface and demands of the feedforward-feedback loop. It was noticed that the distribution of the visual sampling of the feedforward and feedback during the sessions differed between subjects and within subjects as therapy sessions progressed. This could be an interesting area of investigation in future studies to better understand how adults learn in a non-instructional and sensory manner. This paradigm needs to be tested further with a larger study and a 30–60 day follow-up to evaluate retention of brain-muscle strategies learnt and further generalizations to other functional activities. Two larger, case-controlled studies are underway presently with sub-acute and chronic phase patients to understand how the transition from hospital to home-based therapy may be executed using the SynPhNe system, and the effect on outcomes and independence.

5. Conclusion

Training to relax specific muscles adequately and in a timely manner during therapy using a feedforward-feedback loop, instead of practicing repetitive muscle contraction alone, may help re-learn movement and daily functional activities in stroke subjects who have "plateaued" and not responding to further therapy.

Simultaneous activation-relaxation training of agonist-antagonist not only facilitated improvement of functional abilities but was also well tolerated by all subjects and did not cause them to get overwhelmed by the number of feedforward and feedback elements on the computer screen. This indicated that despite the challenges brought on by stroke, patients with impairments can still leverage their sensory learning abilities in an exploratory and then goal-directed manner while attempting to regain spatial and temporal aspects of movement and function of the upper limb. Thus, they appeared to be able to re-boot how they learnt in a sensory manner as babies using the feedforward-feedback modality. A wearable device such as the SynPhNe system may, therefore, help leverage neuroplasticity and act as a key complement to conventional therapy. Being patient-led and requiring reduced therapist supervision, it can effectively augment therapy hours at home or in the community, thus holding the promise of making daily therapy accessible and affordable to all.

Acknowledgements

The research was funded by the National Research Foundation POC Grant and Singapore-MIT Alliance for Research and Technology (SMART) Innovation Grant, both in Singapore. Our thanks also go out to the subjects who participated and the clinical teams at Tan Tock Seng Hospital and National University Hospital, Singapore.

Conflict of interest

Subhasis Banerji and John Heng are founders and inventors of the SynPhNe system. While providing technical support and supervision to the studies, they were blinded to pre- and post-clinical assessment of subjects.

Daphne Menezes and Ponvignesh Ponnusamy are current employees of Synphne Pte. Ltd., Singapore. Daphne Menezes assisted the clinical study team as a trainer in the SynPhNe system and observer of therapy sessions. Ponvignesh Ponnusamy assisted with software programming and user interface development only. Both were blinded to pre- and post-clinical assessment of subjects.

The other authors have no conflict of interest.

Author details

Subhasis Banerji[1*], John Heng[2], Effie Chew[3], Christopher Wee Keong Kuah[4], Ling Zhao[3], Soh Yan Ming[4], Daphne Menezes[1] and Ponvignesh Ponnusamy[1]

1 SynPhNe Pte. Ltd, Singapore

2 Nanyang Technological University, Singapore

3 National University of Singapore, Singapore

4 Tan Tock Seng Hospital, Singapore

*Address all correspondence to: subhasis@synphne.com

References

[1] van Putten MJ, Tavy DL. Continuous quantitative EEG monitoring in hemispheric stroke patients using the brain symmetry index. Stroke. 2004;**35**(11):2489-2492

[2] Kollen B, Kwakkel G, Lindeman E. Functional recovery after stroke: A review of current developments in stroke rehabilitation research. Reviews on Recent Clinical Trials. 2006;**1**(1):75-80

[3] Kwakkel G, Kollen BJ, Krebs HI. Effects of robot-assisted therapy on upper limb recovery after stroke: A systematic review. Neurorehabilitation and Neural Repair. 2008;**22**(2):111-121

[4] Timmermans AA, Seelen HA, Willmann RD, Kingma H. Technology-assisted training of arm-hand skills in stroke: Concepts on reacquisition of motor control and therapist guidelines for rehabilitation technology design. Journal of Neuroengineering and Rehabilitation. 2009;**6**:1

[5] Loureiro RCV, Collin CF, Harwin WS. Robot aided therapy: Challenges ahead for upper limb stroke rehabilitation. In: Proc 5th Intl Conf on Disability, Virtual Reality and Assoc Technologies; 20-22 September 2004; Oxford, UK. Reading: The University of Reading; 2004. pp. 33-39

[6] Bach-y-Rita P. Plasticity of the nervous system: Importance in medical rehabilitation practice. In: Clinical Advances in Physical Medicine and Rehabilitation. Washington DC: Pan American Health Organization; 1991. pp. 58-78

[7] Taub E. Somatosensory deafferentation in research with monkeys: Implications for rehabilitation medicine. In: Behavioural Psychology and Rehabilitation Medicine: Clinical Applications. New York: Williams & Wilkins; 1980. pp. 371-401

[8] Weiss P, Jeannerod M. Getting a grasp on coordination. News in Physiological Sciences. 1998;**13**:70-75

[9] Haken H, Kelso JA, Bunz H. A theoretical model of phase transitions in human hand movements. Biological Cybernetics. 1985;**51**(5):347-356

[10] Bernstein N. The Coordination and Regulation of Movements. New York: Pergamon Press; 1967

[11] Campolo D, Accoto D, Formica D, Guglielmelli E. Intrinsic constraints of neural origin: Assessment and application to rehabilitation robotics. IEEE Transactions on Robotics. 2009;**25**(3):492-501

[12] Gelfand IM, Latash ML. On the problem of adequate language in motor control. Motor Control. 1998;**2**(4):306-313

[13] Bhat N, Bhat K. Coronary disease and congestive heart disorder. In: Handbook of Mind-Body Medicine for Primary Care. Thousand Oaks, CA: Sage Publications, Inc; 2003. pp. 249-258

[14] Ornish D, Brown SE, Scherwitz LW, Billings JH, Armstrong WT, Ports TA, et al. Can lifestyle changes reverse coronary heart disease? The lifestyle heart trial. Lancet. 1990;**336**(8708):129-133

[15] Siegel BS. Love, Medicine and Miracles: Lessons Learned about Self-Healing from a Surgeon's Experience with Exceptional Patients. New York: William Morrow Paperbacks; 1998

[16] Wulf G. Self-controlled practice enhances motor learning: Implications for physiotherapy. Physiotherapy. 2007;**93**(2):96-101

[17] Schallert T, Woodlee MT, Fleming SM. Experimental focal ischemic injury:

Behavior-brain interactions and issues of animal handling and housing. ILAR Journal. 2003;**44**(2):130-143

[18] Bach-y-Rita P. Thoughts on the role of the mind in recovery from brain damage. In: Machinery of the Mind. Boston, MA: Birkhäuser; 1990. pp. 353-359

[19] Taub E, Miller NE, Novack TA, Cook EW 3rd, Fleming WC, Nepomuceno CS, et al. Technique to improve chronic motor deficit after stroke. Archives of Physical Medicine and Rehabilitation. 1993;**74**(4):347-354

[20] Sakata K, Martinowich K, Woo NH, Schloesser RJ, Jimenez DV, Ji Y, et al. Role of activity-dependent BDNF expression in hippocampal-prefrontal cortical regulation of behavioral perseverance. Proceedings of the National Academy of Sciences of the United States of America. 2003;**110**(37):15103-15108

[21] Kleim JA, Jones TA, Schallert T. Motor enrichment and induction of brain plasticity before or after brain injury. Neurochemical Research. 2003;**28**(11):1757-1769

[22] Velasquez JD, 1998. When robots weep: Emotional memories and decision-making. In: Proc 15th Natl Conf on Artificial Intelligence; 27-29 July 1998; Madison, USA. California: American Association for Artificial Intelligence; 1998. pp. 70-75

[23] Smith L, Gasser M. The development of embodied cognition: Six lessons from babies. Artificial Life. 2006;**11**(1-2):13-29

[24] Taylor JB. My Stroke of Insight: A Brain Scientist's Personal Journey. England: Hodder Paperbacks; 2009

[25] Edelman G. Neural Darwinism. New York: Basic Books; 1987

[26] Elman JL. Learning and development in neural networks: The importance of starting small. Cognition. 1993;**48**(1):71-99

[27] Ballard D, Hayhoe MM, Pook PK, Rao RP. Deictic codes for the embodiment of cognition. The Behavioral and Brain Sciences. 1997;**20**(4):723-742

[28] Baldwin D. Early referential understanding: Infants' ability to recognize referential acts for what they are. Developmental Psychology. 1993;**29**(5):832-843

[29] DeLoache JS. The symbol mindedness of young children. In: Child Psychology in Retrospect and Prospect: In Celebration of the 75th Anniversary of the Institute of Child Development: The Minnesota Symposia on Child Psychology. Vol. 32. Mahwah, NJ: L. Erlbaum Associates; 2002. pp. 73-101

[30] Deci EL, Eghrari H, Patrick BC, Leone DR. Facilitating internalization: The self-determination theory perspective. Journal of Personality. 1994;**62**(1):119-142

[31] Ito K, Doi M, Kondo T. Feed-Forward Adaptation to a Varying Dynamic Environment During Reaching Movements. J. Robot. Mechatron. 2007;**19**(4):474-481

[32] Meilink A, Hemmen B, Seelen HA, Kwakkel G. Impact of EMG-triggered neuromuscular stimulation of the wrist and finger extensors of the paretic hand after stroke: A systematic review of the literature. Clinical Rehabilitation. 2008;**22**(4):291-305

[33] Caspers S, Zilles K, Laird AR, Eickhoff SB. ALE meta-analysis of action observation and imitation in the human brain. NeuroImage. 2010;**50**(3):1148-1167

[34] Hecht H, Vogt S, Prinz W. Motor learning enhances perceptual judgement: A case for action-perception

transfer. Psychological Research. 2001;**65**(1):3-14

[35] Mehlink WE, Wrubel J, Daubenmier JJ, Price CJ, Kerr CE, Silow T, et al. Body awareness: A phenomenological inquiry into the common ground of mind-body therapies. Philosophy, Ethics, and Humanities in Medicine. 2011;**6**:6

[36] Heng J, Banerji S. Low usage of intelligent technologies for the aged: New initiatives to bridge the digital divide. In: Digital Literacy: Concepts, Methodologies, Tools, and Applications. Hershey, PA: IGI Global; 2010. pp. 135-153

[37] Heng J, Banerji S. A step towards multi-level human interface devices: A system that responds to EEG/SEMG triggers. International Journal of Biomechatronics and Biomedical Robotics. 2010;**1**(2):93-98

[38] Kaplanis PA, Pattichis CS, Hadjileontiadis LJ, Roberts VC. Surface EMG analysis on normal subjects based on isometric voluntary contraction. Journal of Electromyography and Kinesiology. 2009;**19**(1):157-171

[39] Banerji S, Heng J, Ponvignesh PS, Menezes D. Augmenting rehabilitation after stroke: A flexible platform for combining multi-channel biofeedback with FES, converging clinical and engineering research on neurorehabilitation I. Biosystems and Biorobotics. 2012;**1**:259-263

[40] Platz T, Pinkowski C, van Wijck F, Kim IH, di Bella P, Johnson G. Reliability and validity of arm function assessment with standardized guidelines for the fugl-meyer test, action research arm test and box and block test: A multicentre study. Clinical Rehabilitation. 2005;**19**(4):404-411

[41] Page SJ, Fulk GD, Boyne P. Clinically important differences for the upper-extremity fugl-meyer scale in people with minimal to moderate impairment due to chronic stroke. Physical Therapy. 2012;**92**(6):791-798

[42] Van der Lee JH, De Groot V, Beckerman H, Wagenaar RC, Lankhorst GJ, Bouter LM. The intra- and interrater reliability of the action research arm test: A practical test of upper extremity function in patients with stroke. Archives of Physical Medicine and Rehabilitation. 2001;**82**(1):14-19

[43] Wagner JM, Dromerick AW, Sahrmann SA, Lang CE. Upper extremity muscle activation during recovery of reaching in subjects with post-stroke hemiparesis. Clinical Neurophysiology. 2007;**118**(1):164-176

[44] Mehrholz J, Platz T, Kugler J, Pohl M. Electromechanical and robot-assisted arm training for improving arm function and activities of daily living after stroke. In J. Mehrholz (Ed.), Cochrane Database of Systematic Reviews. Chichester, UK: John Wiley & Sons, Ltd. 2008 (p. CD006876). DOI: 10.1002/14651858.CD006876.pub2

[45] Hesse S, Schulte-Tigges G, Konrad M, Bardeleben A, Werner C. Robot assisted arm trainer for the passive and active practice of bilateral forearm and wrist movements in hemiparetic subjects. Archives of Physical Medicine and Rehabilitation. 2003;**84**(6):915-920

[46] Pomeroy VM, King IM, Pollock A, Baily-Hallam A, Langhorne P. Electrostimulation for promoting recovery of movement or functional ability after stroke: Systematic review and meta analysis. Stroke. 2006;**37**:2441-2442

[47] Broeks JG, Lankhorst GJ, Rumping K, Prevo AJ. The long term outcome of arm function after stroke: Results of a follow-up study. Disability and Rehabilitation. 1999;**21**(8):357-364

[48] Gordon NF, Gulanick M, Costa F, Fletcher G, Franklin BA, Roth EJ, et al. Physical activity and exercise recommendations for stroke survivors: An American Heart Association Scientific Statement from the Council of Clinical Cardiology, Subcommittee on Exercise, Cardiac Rehabilitation and Prevention; the Council on Cardiovascular Nursing; the Council on Nutrition, Physical Activity and Metabolism; and the Stroke Council. Stroke. 2004;**35**(5):1230-1240

[49] Banerji S, Heng J, Banerjee A, Menezes D, Kumar R. Delivering remote rehabilitation at home: An integrated physio-neuro approach to effective and user friendly wearable devices. Converging clinical and engineering research on neurorehabilitation II. Biosystems and Biorobotics. 2016;**15**:1097-1101

Section 4

Assistive Systems

Chapter 8

An Embedded Gait Analysis System for CNS Injury Patients

Gilbert Pradel, Tong Li, Didier Pradon and Nicolas Roche

Abstract

Clinical evaluation of CNS injury patients before and after treatment is an essential step in gait rehabilitation. Medical care of gait disturbance for stroke patients is based on different treatments based on clinical and functional evaluations. Evaluation of gait aims at characterizing the motor performance to provide clinicians with information on the patient's organizational or performance status and to allow them to consider the most appropriate treatment options. A 3D instrumented gait analysis system allows quantification of several parameters at each instant of walking but does not represent gait in daily life conditions. The absence of devices usable in daily life situation constitutes a lack pointed out by clinical practitioners and is at the origin of this work. In the following are described the design and implementation of a wireless embedded system for the collection of spatiotemporal parameters of pathological gait in everyday life. Algorithms estimate joint angles, step length, and gait events and automatically partition data into gait cycles. Experiments have been carried out to accurately evaluate the joint angles, the precision of sensor synchronization, the precision of gait event detection, and the robustness in the case of pathological walk. Comparisons with references given by the 3D instrumented gait analysis system are detailed.

Keywords: CNS injury people, stroke patients, gait analysis, spatiotemporal gait parameters, gait event detection, embedded systems

1. Introduction

Stroke, caused by an effusion of the blood inside the brain tissue (hemorrhage) or by an interruption of the blood supply (ischemia), leads to motor impairments and disorders of the higher functions (e.g. negligence and anosognosia), sensorial and sensitive [1–3].

On the motor plan, the lesion of the central nervous system generates a pyramidal syndrome mainly characterized by a loss of motor selectivity, alteration of motor command, and a muscle over-activity accompanied by exaggeration of the stretch reflex commonly called spasticity. Although 50–80% of the patients recover a locomotor capacity [1, 4], they reported that, due to gait alteration, they lost a lot of autonomy in daily life activities [5–7].

Human gait is a complex phenomenon that must ensure the inter-limb coordination rotation of multiple segments in order to maintain equilibrium during motion [3]. It can be described as a series of segmental rotations of the lower limbs in order to ensure the displacement of the body. These series of cyclic movements can be split into different phases grouped together in a gait cycle. Hemiplegic patients' gait

 IntechOpen

differs from those of healthy people concerning different points like performance and organization. The main anomalies observed in this population are an alteration of spatiotemporal and kinematic parameters. Therapeutic management and prospective follow-up take into account these two points.

Medical care of gait disturbance in stroke patients use different treatments based on clinical evaluation and functional evaluation. Evaluation of the stroke patient's gait aims at characterizing the motor performance to provide clinicians with information on the patient's organizational or performance status and to allow them to consider the most appropriate treatment options.

In the same way, after applying these different therapeutic approaches, the evaluation allows the therapist to determine the effectiveness of the latter in relation to the fixed objective. Among the different methods for evaluating gait, the most commonly used to know the patient's organization during walking are the Functional Gait Assessment (FGA) and the 3D instrumented Gait Analysis (3D-GA).

There are different types of functional tests that can be used in varying scenarios to evaluate the locomotion of hemiparetic patients. Here, we just list some of the most used tests:

- The 5- or 10-m walking test: timed walk on a set distance (5 or 10 m) with spontaneous or maximum speed. With this test, the mean of speed, cadence, and step length could be determined.

- The 6-minute walk test: assesses the maximum distance walked during 6 minutes over a 30 m [8, 9] walkway to determine the average walk speed.

- The Timed Up and GO test: the patient is asked to rise from a chair, walk 3 m, turn, walk back to the chair and sit down. It can be used to assess walking speed, functional mobility, walking balance, and postural transitions.

The FGAs are performed under the situations close to those of the patient's daily life but do not provide all the parameters characterizing walking. They do not allow observing the evolution of all the parameters and also limit the number of measurable parameters; their measurement is generally not precise because it is too qualitative.

The 3D-GA provides the clinician with all the quantitative information on the state of organization of the musculoskeletal system during the execution of the locomotor task by means of the kinematic, kinetic, and spatiotemporal parameters of the gait. A 3D-GA system uses the absolute three-dimensional location of the object moving relative to a system reference also fixed. It can be typically of optoelectronic type (Motion Analysis, Vicon, Optitrack, Qualisys, Saga, Codamotion, etc.). The patient, equipped with reflective markers located on anatomical points, walks in an environment equipped with optoelectronic cameras that record the displacement of the markers, of a platform of force to detect the events of the gait cycle. A complex post processing on the recorded information extracts the locomotor parameters. This test can only be performed in a hospital environment with limitations due to the size of the environment and its duration.

The walk of the patient in the hospital environment, equipped with these reflective markers, may be not representative of his/her locomotion in everyday life: the distance is too short, the ground is horizontal without asperities, and the trajectory is very often rectilinear. When using a treadmill, the start and stop phases are delicate for the patient's balance. Also, finding a device providing information on walking is a necessity.

An embedded wearable motion analysis system uses a set of sensors worn on the body of the person to measure locomotion parameters. The system must be energy efficient, light, and compact and must not interfere with the patient's natural locomotion so that it can be used in patients' everyday life. Information provided by the embedded system must be similar to those delivered by 3D-GA systems.

This chapter describes the wireless embedded system for acquiring the locomotor parameters of a stroke person. This system is designed to be used out of hospital environment (i.e. in the patient's daily life). This system is coupled to a gait event detection device to isolate walking cycles. The results of the experiments performed are compared to those provided by the 3D-GA in order to test the accuracy and robustness of the proposed system.

2. Changes in hemiplegic gait

2.1 Changes in spatiotemporal parameters of the gait cycle

The gait cycle, normal or pathologic, is divided into eight sub-phases: initial contact, loading response, midstance, terminal stance, pre-swing, initial swing, mid swing, and late swing [10, 11]. If the full cycle is normalized to 100%, then the stance phase (between initial contact (IC) event and final contact (FC) event) represents 60% and the swing phase 40%. This normalization makes it possible to compare the results of different studies or different populations.

The spatiotemporal parameters are often used to describe and characterize the locomotion [3, 10]. **Figure 1** illustrates the definition of the spatial parameters like step width, step length, and stride length.

The following are the temporal parameters:

- Duration of the different sub-phases, expressed in percentage
- Cadence in number of steps per minute
- Lengths of the step and the stride
- Gait speed, which is the product of the cadence per step length in m/s

If, for a healthy subject, the durations of the sub-phases in a cycle are symmetrical for the left and the right sides, it is not the case for a stroke patient. In that case, the duration of the stance phase and its percentage of the gait cycle decrease for the affected lower limb compared to the healthy subject [12–16]. Moreover, the duration of the single support phase of the paretic side is decreased compared to the healthy side. The spontaneous gait speed can be considered as a significant element that traduces patients' ability to walk [10]. Similarly, different studies [17, 18]

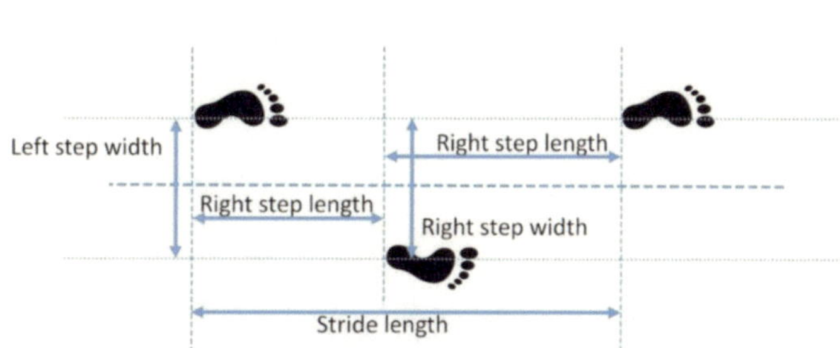

Figure 1.
Spatial parameters.

showed that the cadence of the stroke patients is decreased compared to those of the healthy subject whatever their gait speed.

2.2 Changes in joint kinematic parameters

The modifications of spatiotemporal parameters observed during gait of stroke patients are mainly caused by kinematic and kinetic alterations [19]. Global motor organization is given by the kinematic parameters, a segment rotation is characterized in function of the adjacent one, and joint angles are the main elements allowing the understanding of the gait. **Figure 2** illustrates the definition of joint angles of the lower limb.

2.2.1 Changes in movement at the hip

The joint angle of the hip is defined as the relative angle between the pelvis and the femur. The flexion/extension of the hip occurs in the sagittal plane. The flexion of the hip propels the thigh toward the anterior surface of the body. In contrast, the extension of the hip throws the thigh toward the posterior surface of the body.

For the healthy subject, at the beginning of a cycle, the hip is in flexion. During the single support phase, the hip performs an extension. At the end of propulsion, the angle of the hip reaches a maximum extension of about −10°. During the oscillating phase, the maximum value of hip flexion can reach +45°.

Usually, a stroke patient exhibits both an insufficient hip flexion and a limitation of the hip extension, [20] which contribute to the decrease of the step length and of the gait speed.

2.2.2 Changes in movement at the knee

The joint angle of the knee, defined as the relative angle between the tight and the shank, is close to +10° for the healthy subject at the beginning of a gait cycle. During the single support phase, this angle increases to a first maximum amplitude of about +20° and then decreases. At the beginning of the oscillating phase, the knee flexes quickly to prepare the oscillation of the body. We then observe a second local maximum with a value that can reach +60° followed by an extension.

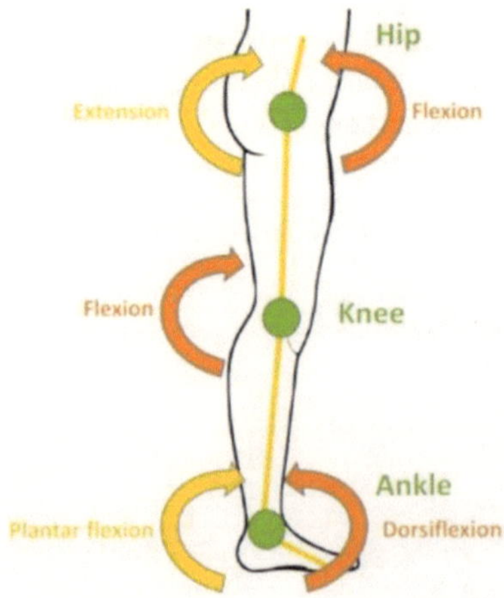

Figure 2.
Definition of the joint angles for the lower limb.

For the stroke patient, the presence of a hyper-extension at the beginning of the single support phase due to the spasticity of the triceps surae or a decrease of peak knee flexion in swing phase is called stiff knee gait mainly due to a spasticity of the rectus femoris muscle.

2.2.3 Changes in movement at the ankle

The ankle joint angle is defined as the relative angle between the shank and the foot, the foot being considered as a single rigid segment. The dorsiflexion of the ankle in the sagittal plane traduces a flexion of the foot. In contrast, plantar flexion comes from a flexion of the foot.

During the gait cycle, the evolution of ankle angle is composed by three steps:

- During the initial double contact, the heel touches the ground with the foot in neutral position (0°).
- Then, the ankle makes a plantar flexion. When the entire foot is in contact with the ground, the ankle plantar flexion is about +10°.
- After this step, the foot makes a dorsiflexion to reach a peak whose value is about +20°.
- The last step corresponds to the toe off. The ankle makes, firstly, a plantar flexion and, secondly, a dorsiflexion.

In stroke patients, a plantar flexion is often observed either during the initial double contact or during the single support phase or the swing phase. This decrease of dorsiflexion can be explained by a spasticity of the triceps surae muscle. This phenomenon is often associated with a reduction of the propulsive force and a deficit of the gait velocity [21, 22].

2.3 Discussion

During an evaluation of the therapeutic management, the following are considered:

- The relative segmental (articular kinematics) and the absolute displacements (segmental kinematics)
- The movements of the segmental and/or global center of mass by using anthropometric data, kinetics, forces, moments, and articular powers by coupling dynamometric sensors (force platform type)
- Electromyographic muscular activities

To allow appropriate management of the stoke patient, the 3D-GA system, considered de facto as the "gold standard," and the FGAs are the most used methods. However, the costs as well as the complexity of the use of optoelectronic 3D-GA systems reduce the use of this assessment of gait disturbance of patients with stroke sequelae to a limited number of laboratories/hospitals compared to the actual demand of patients.

The studies presented in the following describe the design and implementation of a wireless embedded system for collecting gait parameters of pathological gait in everyday life.

3. Recording of gait parameters by wireless wearable system

The main objective at the base of the approach is the study of the signals from the sensors during walking and the implementation of the posture estimation algorithm. This section describes the architecture of the realized prototype as well as the algorithm used to estimate the posture. The flexions and extensions of the segments estimated by the prototype are compared with the measurements from the 3D-GA system considered as a reference. The results of this comparison will be shown in the experimentation section.

3.1 System architecture

Different types of noninvasive sensors are able to measure the gait kinematics, such as magnetic sensors, goniometers, and inertial measurement units (IMU). These IMUs, consisting of sensors, measure the acceleration, the angular velocity, and the terrestrial magnetic field density around the sensor in the orthonormal coordinate system bound to the sensors. This information is used to estimate the orientation of the human body segments on which the sensors are placed. The joint angles are then calculated based on the orientations of the segments.

The IMU and compass sensor based on MEMS (Micro Electro Mechanical System) technology allow the design of miniaturized wireless sensors respecting the constraints of energy consumption, compactness, and cost. Therefore, the system uses MEMS IMU and compass sensor to capture the movement of lower limb segments.

The system comprises at least seven sensor nodes as shown in **Figure 3**. Each node is built around the System-on-Chip (SoC) Nrf51822 from Nordic Semiconductors. It offers many low-power wireless communication options, including ESB and Bluetooth Low Energy (BLE) protocols. The inertial sensor used is the MPU6050 from Invensense. This IMU integrates a 3D accelerometer and a 3D gyrometer. A 3D magnetometer is used to measure the Earth's magnetic field. Measurements carried out by the sensors are processed by the onboard SoC to estimate their orientations in real time.

A coordinator node supports the synchronization of the sensor nodes, the recording of the data coming from the sensor nodes on a SD card, and the management of the various functions of the sensor node (connection/disconnection,

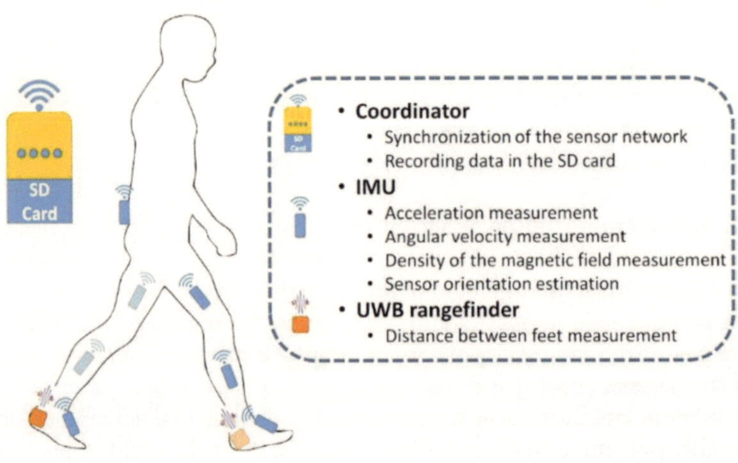

Figure 3.
System organization and sensor placement.

calibration, and power on/off). The sensor nodes wait for synchronization with the coordinator and then transmit the data to it. This wireless distributed system architecture provides great system flexibility and greatly improves its ease of use.

3.2 Constraints related to the use of a wireless device

The wireless transmission protocol, in addition to being energy efficient, must have enough bandwidth to transmit measurements in accordance with the required sampling frequency. The protocol must allow synchronization of the clocks of the various sensors to have the same time reference. Clock synchronization, imperative in our application, allows separate systems to have the smallest possible difference between their subjective times whatever the factors that can modify the time reference [23].

Candidate technologies, such as WIFI (IEEE 802.11), ZigBee (IEEE 8.2.15.4), Bluetooth classic, BLE, GSM, 3G, and LTE, have not been selected because either they do not allow a precise synchronization of the sensor nodes, or they do not provide the desired throughput or limit the number of nodes. The chosen protocol, ESB, is a proprietary low energy consumption protocol proposed by Nordic Semiconductor with a bit rate of 2 Mbps. It reaches a transmission speed of 1.2 Mbps. It supports broadcast functionality to synchronize clocks.

Without the time synchronization, the time shift between sensors may achieve 144 ms after 1 hour of measurement using a clock with accuracy equal to 20 ppm. Synchronization accuracy tests were performed. The synchronization RMSE calculated during the last minute after 1 hour of recording is equal to 18.2 μs. During the test, the maximum clock offset between two sensor nodes is 37.6 μs.

The average of the sampling period of the system, i.e. the duration between two synchronizations, equals 9.1 ms with a standard deviation of 1.1 ms. The acquisition frequency of system locomotive parameters can reach 109 Hz.

3.3 Joint angle reckoning

Each sensor node has its own reference system. It is then necessary to define a suitable coordinate system to describe the orientation of a lower limb's segment. Two coordinate systems are used in this application. One system is fixed to the earth and may be considered for the purpose of segment of human motion analysis to be an inertial coordinate system. The other coordinate system is local to the IMU and is referred to as a body coordinate system. The attitude of an object can be represented in different ways [24]. Euler angles, rotation matrix, and quaternion are the most used methods. Quaternion is difficult to understand but compared to the two other representation methods, it requires less memory and calculation capabilities. It avoids the problem of Gimbal lock that appears in Euler angle representation. The quaternion representation is used in this application. A complete description of the use of quaternions for articular angle calculation between two segments and the transformation of the local coordinate system to the terrestrial reference is described in [24, 25].

Data captured by IMU and magnetometer are processed in real time with the algorithm executed by the onboard SoC to estimate sensor attitude. This algorithm uses a numerical integration to compute the angle from the angular velocity provided by the gyrometer. This numerical integration inevitably introduces a drift in addition to the calculation approximation error. To correct this drift which accumulates over time, the information provided by the accelerometer and the magnetometer have been merged according to the onboard algorithm. The detail of this algorithm is described in [26, 27].

Finally, tests in static and dynamic conditions show that the adopted method is effective to compensate the drift of the gyrometer during walk. The quality of estimation is related to the conditions of use of the sensor (vibration, percussion, and external accelerations experienced during a long time…). Nevertheless, if the IMU works on a limit condition for a very long duration, the risk of incorrect estimated value remains present. In the case of gait in everyday life, these conditions occur periodically, but not during a long time, the precision of estimated values remains in acceptable limits.

Thanks to this system, it is possible to calculate the joint angles of the lower limb in real time and to record them in an everyday life environment.

3.4 Experiments

The experiments are carried out in a gait analysis laboratory equipped with 3D-GA system, considered as reference, to evaluate the accuracy of the proposed system. Three healthy subjects and two hemiparetic patients have been experimented with wearing markers for 3D-GA system and the wearable system. The hemiparetic patients perform 6 times a course of 8 m with self-select comfortable speed. The 3D-GA system capture area is approximately 6 m × 3 m; this limits the recording time. To evaluate the reliability of the proposed system for a longer duration, it has been decided to practice the experiments on a treadmill. To avoid the difficulties encountered by hemiparetic patients, especially when starting the carpet, only the healthy subjects have been asked to walk on the treadmill. The healthy persons have been asked to walk on the treadmill for 1 minute. The speed of the treadmill is set at 4 km/h.

Figure 4 shows the evolution of joint angles of a hemiparetic patient during walking on flat terrain (right side in blue and left side in red). The signals of both systems have a great similarity in shape. There is no time shift, and the differences between the signals from the two systems are limited.

Figure 5 illustrates the changes in joint angles in the sagittal plane of a healthy person while walking on a treadmill. The joint angles estimated by the proposed system are the continuous line signals and those measured by the 3D-GA system are in dashed line. The figure shows joint angles in a 10-second window of a 1-minute recording. As for the signals observed on the hemiplegic patient, the signals of both systems have a great similarity in shape. The two systems are well synchronized. The differences between the signals from the two systems are limited.

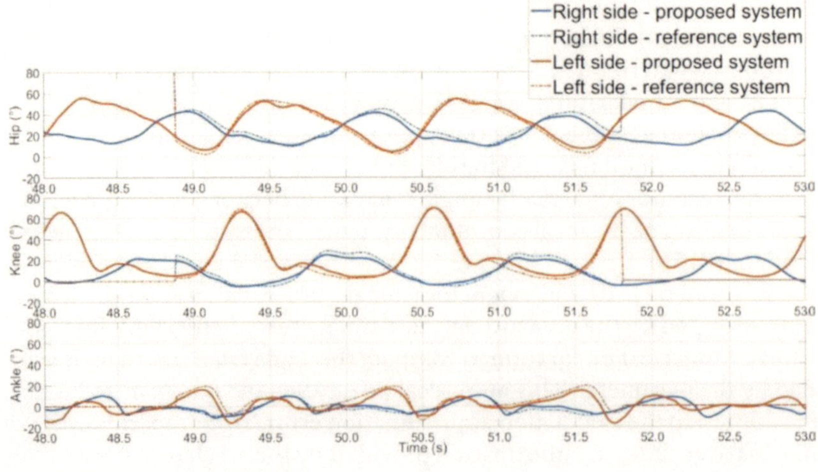

Figure 4.
Joint angles of a hemiparetic subject.

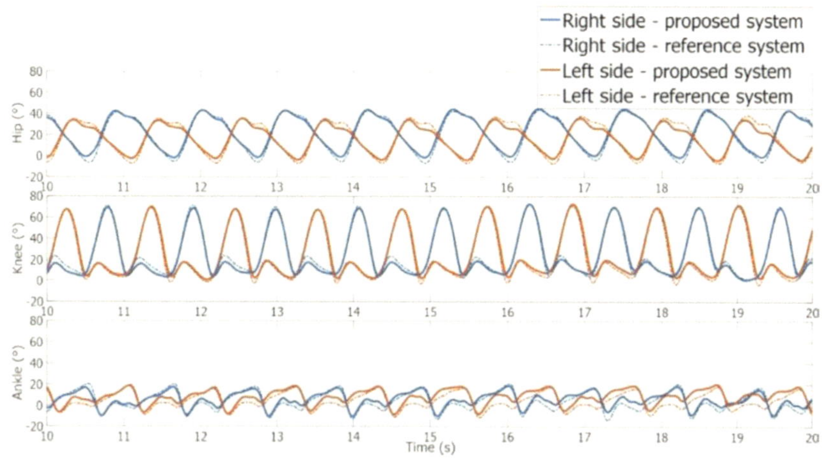

Figure 5.
Joint angles of a healthy subject during treadmill walking.

Table 1 illustrates the accuracy of the wearable system compared to the 3D-GA system. Root mean square error (RMSE) allows us to observe the difference of each sample between the two systems. The correlation coefficient (CC) allows us to evaluate the similarity of the shapes of the signals measured by the two systems. The RMSEs of joint angles estimated with respect to the reference system are between 2.4° and 4.0° for healthy persons. The CCs of healthy subjects are between 0.89 and 0.99. The signals of the hemiparetic patients have RMSEs between 3.1° and 3.6° and CCs between 0.89 and 0.99.

Figure 6 illustrates the correlation and concordance of the joint angles measured by the two systems. The coefficient of determination (r^2) equals 0.97. The lower limits of agreement (95%) equal −4.8° and the upper limits of agreement (95%) equal 7.6°.

3.5 Discussion

Comparisons between the results of the embedded system and the reference show that the joint angles measured by the embedded system have limited differences compared to the reference system. The RMSE of the proposed system is between 2.4° and 4.0°. The signal shapes of both systems have great similarities. The CC of the signals between two systems is between 0.89 and 0.99.

		Joint angle					
		Ankle		Knee		Hip	
		RMSE (°)	CC	RMSE (°)	CC	RMSE (°)	CC
Hemiparetic subject	1	3.6	0.90	3.3	0.98	3.5	0.98
	2	3.2	0.89	3.4	0.98	3.1	0.97
Average		3.4	0.90	3.3	0.98	3.3	0.98
Healthy subject	1	4.0	0.90	3.1	0.99	3.3	0.97
	2	3.9	0.89	3.0	0.99	2.4	0.99
	3	3.4	0.92	3.2	0.99	3.2	0.98
Average		3.8	0.90	3.1	0.99	3.0	0.98

Table 1.
Comparison between the proposed system and the 3D-GA system.

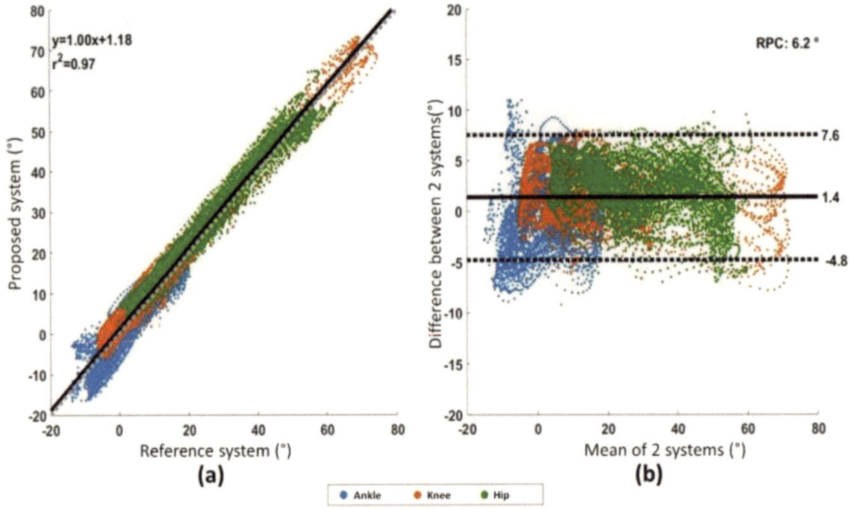

Figure 6.
Correlation (a) and Bland-Altman plot (b).

From the results of the comparison (**Table 1**), **Figures 6** and 7, the largest RMSE and the smallest CC are observed for the joint angles of the ankles. Three sources may induce these errors: percussion during walking, centripetal acceleration, and the cross-talk effect [28]. During the walk, the main percussions occur when the foot contacts the ground. Percussions influence the measurements of accelerometers and gyrometers; the filtering process used to reduce these influences does not fully eliminate them. Measurement errors can also be introduced by the cross-talk effect. During a straight walk, the ankles have more degrees of freedom than other joints. When positioning a sensor, there can be misalignments between the sensor and the segment of the human body. The consequence is that the movements in the planes other than the sagittal plane are combined in the measure. This problem can be solved by adding a calibration phase to align the sensor and human body [29]. This problem will be considered in a future study.

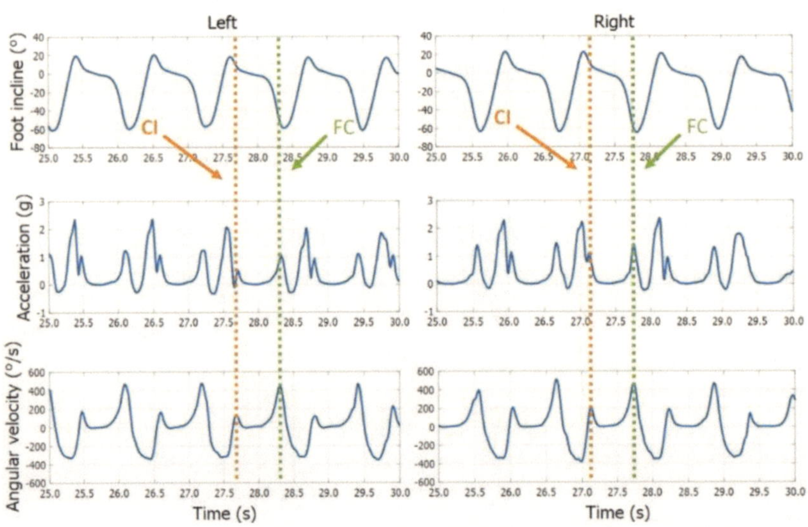

Figure 7.
IMU signals and gait events of a healthy subject.

To conclude this section, despite the lack of a precise calibration process, the embedded system provides an estimate of the joint angles close to the references, which validates both the architecture and the data processing algorithm.

Data captured by the system are organized in time series; this does not allow to analyze or compare inter or between patients. In gait analysis, locomotion data are often partitioned with gait event and normalized in gait cycle to compare with each other. The size of data captured in everyday life condition is often huge. A method to perform auto-partition is necessary.

4. Determination of gait events

Detection of gait events is a fundamental problem. All captured gait signals should be normalized in gait cycles so that they could be compared between each other. Calculations of spatiotemporal parameters are also based on the timing of gait events. So, the determination of the IC and FC event occurrences is compulsory.

In everyday life conditions, the gait event can be captured whether by measuring the ground reaction force (GRF) or by processing of the signals from IMU.

GRF-based methods use foot switches (force sensitive resistor or mechanical switch) placed under toe and heel to determine IC and FC events. Gait event detection is quite easy with these methods. Due to the GRF, the foot switch state toggles both when the foot contacts the ground (Heel-Strike, IC event) and when the foot leaves the ground (Toe-Off, FC event). These systems are considered as the Gold Standard for normal gait due to their high accuracy.

But in pathological gait, the IC event could not correspond to heel-strike and the FC event not often corresponds to toe-off as in normal gait. For example, with foot drop gait, the IC event may be the moment when the toe starts to contact the ground and FC event is the moment of toe-off. Therefore, it is difficult to place the force sensor for the pathological gait, and this limits its use [30].

Several studies propose real-time or delayed real-time motion detection systems based on the use of acceleration and angular velocity signals of human body segments provided by IMU [30–36]. All the algorithms proposed in these studies consist of a set of rules that make it possible to identify several characteristics in the different gait signals. Currently, in everyday life gait event determination systems, the accelerometer seems to be the most used sensor [37]. The data it provides are often coupled with data from the gyrometer to get more reliable results.

Figure 7 illustrates the acceleration, sagittal angular velocity, and inclination signals of both feet on a healthy subject during normal walking. The signals observed on both feet have almost the same characteristics and shapes. The local extrema of acceleration and angular velocity signals are the most commonly used characteristics for determining gait events (IC and FC) [37]. The accuracy of methods presented in different studies may achieve between 11 and 165 ms [35, 36]. Between 86 and 98% of events are correctly detected for normal gait [37].

Figure 8 shows the acceleration, angular velocity, and inclination signals of the two feet of a hemiparetic patient during a straight walk. Due to the asymmetry of the gait, the acceleration and angular velocity signals are significantly distinct between the healthy side and the paretic side. The amplitudes of the acceleration and angular velocity signals are much lower than those of a healthy person. Local maximum is strongly attenuated, especially the local maximum corresponding to the IC event in the angular velocity signal. In addition, the style of pathological walking varies greatly between stroke persons and there is a significant variability in the shape of the recordings. Given this specificity, it is difficult to use existing

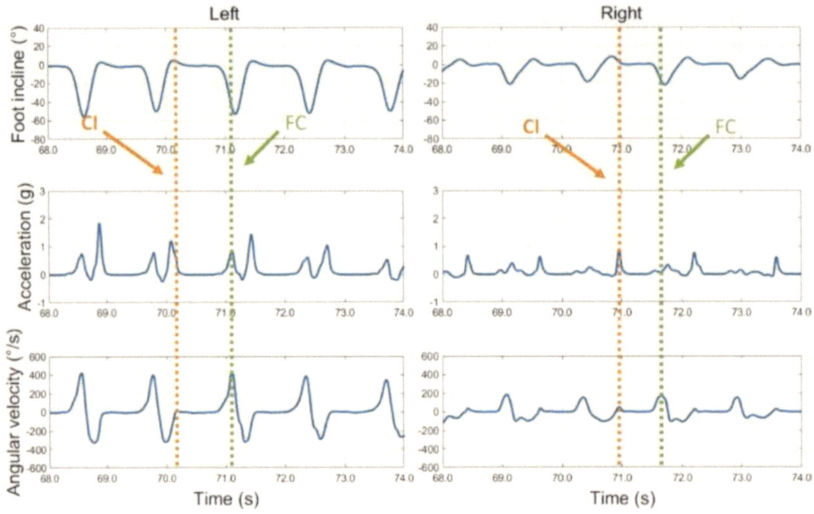

Figure 8.
IMU signals and gait events of a stroke subject.

methods to treat different types of pathological walking. An alternative method is therefore necessary to determine the gait events.

4.1 Proposed method

During walk, the distance between the two feet varies periodically. Assume, at moment t_0, the following situation: both feet are on the ground, right foot forward and left foot back. The beginning of the gait cycle of the right foot is the moment when it touches the ground. The distance between the two feet is maximum, which leads to a local maximum in the feet distance signal. During the single support phase of the right foot, the left foot being in swing phase, the distance between feet decreases until the first local minimum is reached when the left foot passes beside the right foot. This distance then increases to another local maximum when the left foot is on the ground. During the swing phase of the right foot, the second minimum appears when the right foot passes near the left foot. The gait cycle of the right foot ends with increasing distance to the third maximum when the right foot is on the ground. **Figure 9** illustrates the variation in the distance between the two feet during walking of a healthy subject and a stroke subject. Asymmetry in the length of the stroke patients justifies the larger differences in amplitude between adjacent local maximum.

Figure 10 illustrates the variation in the normalized foot distances in the gait cycle of a healthy and of a stroke person during straight walking. The two signals have similar shapes close to the letter 'w'. The signals are composed of three local maxima and two local minima. This phenomenon seeable during the gait of the healthy person is also encountered in pathological walking. The two local maxima located at the beginning and at the end of the gait cycle correspond to the IC event of the same side. The third local maximum located at around 50% of the walking cycle identifies the IC event of the opposite side. The two local minima occur as the feet pass closest to each other. It is observed that the median local maximum on the signal of the healthy people is very close to the point corresponding to 50% of walking cycle. Opposite, because of the gait asymmetry of the hemiparetic patient, the median local maximum is slightly offset from the middle point of the gait cycle.

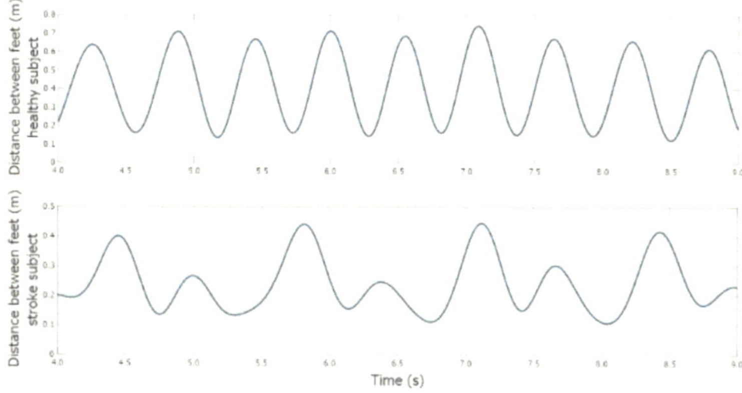

Figure 9.
Distance between feet during walk.

Compared to the acceleration and angular velocity signals, the foot distance signal is simpler to use for the recognition of gait events as the extrema are more significant. The IC event can be highlighted by searching for the local maximum of the foot distance signal.

Figure 11 shows the relationship binding the distance between the two feet and the IC event. In this figure, the blue curve is the relative distance between feet during the walk of the hemiparetic patient. This distance is captured by the 3D-GA system. The red dots correspond to the IC events determined manually by visual inspection. Green triangles are the local maximums of the distance. Local maxima are very close to the IC events determined manually. Feet distance can then be an alternative, simpler, and more robust method than existing ones.

However, local maxima only allow determining that an IC event is produced by a foot. To distinguish, the foot that produces the IC event is the one that has just finished its swing phase, because the opposite foot is in its **support** phase. The acceleration experienced by the foot that produces the IC event must be significantly greater than that of the opposite foot before the IC event. Comparing the accelerations of both feet for a time just before the IC event occurs is the way to identify the foot that produces this event.

After the IC events have been correctly determined, it is then possible to partition and normalize the recording in gait cycles. Between two IC events on the same foot, there must be a FC produced by this foot. Even if the local maxima that correspond to the IC events are attenuated and become undetectable, the local maxima

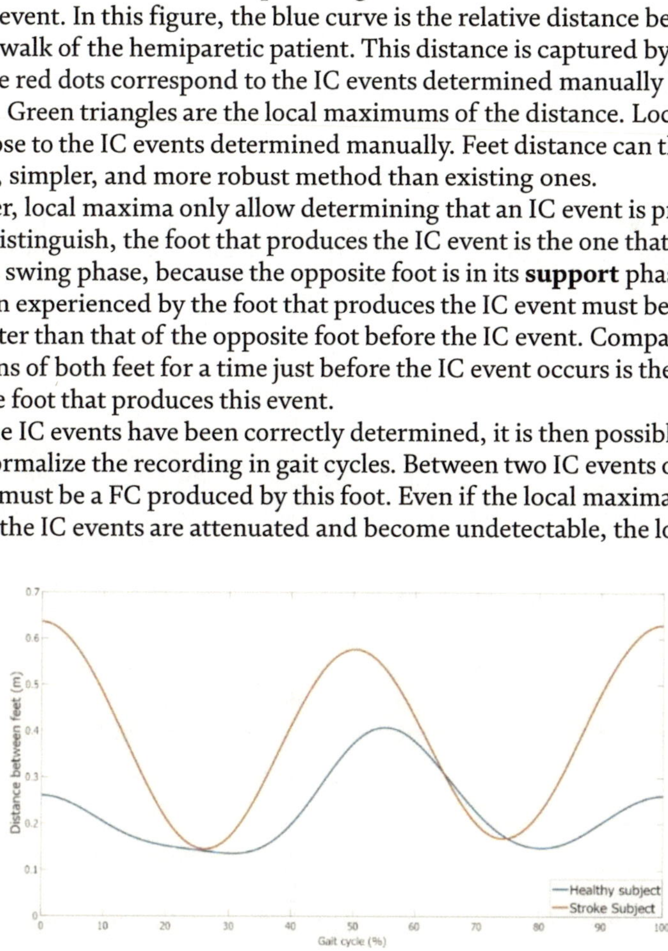

Figure 10.
Distance between feet normalized in gait cycle.

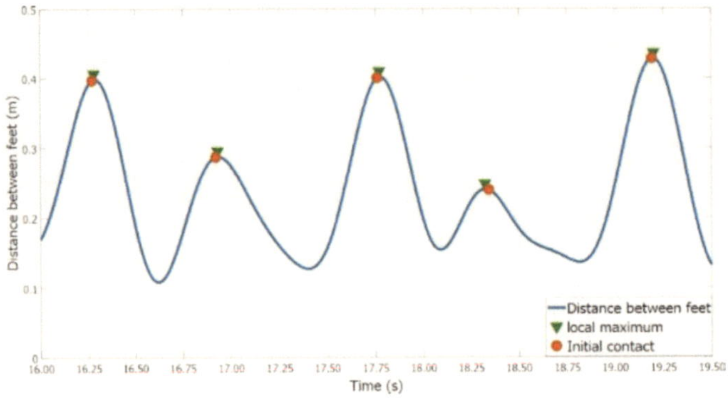

Figure 11.
Relationship between the IC event and the distance between feet.

that correspond to the FC events are still detectable. The method for determining FC using the signal from gyrometer, which is presented in different studies, remains valid [30, 33, 38, 39].

In the following, the new embedded sensor for measuring the relative distance between feet to determine the IC event is described. The data from this new sensor are coupled with data provided by the IMU to determine the FC event. The accuracy of this method is evaluated by comparing the results provided by the proposed system and those given by the 3D-GA system.

The distance between feet can be measured either by measuring the displacements of the two feet independently or by a direct measurement of the distance between the two feet.

Theoretically, the displacement of the foot can be calculated with data from the IMU attached to the foot. After estimating the attitude of the foot, a reference transformation can be made to transform the acceleration measured in the sensor coordinate system to the fixed coordinate system. By double integration on the acceleration of the foot, the three-dimensional displacement of the foot can be reckoned. But unbounded drifts will appear because of the sensor noise and the accumulation of the digital integration error.

Several studies propose different methods based on the algorithm called "zero velocity update" (ZUPT), which aim at reducing this error [40–43]. These methods are based on the detection of the period during which the foot is considered as static or quasi-static according to the information measured by the accelerometer or the gyrometer, supposing that the foot velocity is equal to zero during these periods. These methods limit the error introduced by the first integration applied to the accelerations to obtain the foot speed. However, no correction is applied to the second integration applied to the speed to calculate the displacement. This implies an accumulation of error over time on the calculation of movement of the foot. The study in [44] shows that the same displacement calculated with data from two IMUs does not give the same result. The errors depend on the style of locomotion and the gait speed as well as the type of environment in which walking is performed [45]. For this reason, none of the studies cited use the movements relative between the two feet.

In order to find a solution, a direct real-time measurement of the relative distance of the feet will be made by a wireless rangefinder that will complement the wireless system. The rangefinder measures the distance directly by measuring the time of fight (ToF) of an electromagnetic wave, thus avoiding complex calculations.

4.2 Measurement of feet distance with ultra-wideband (UWB) rangefinder

To determine gait events using foot distance signal, a pair of rangefinder modules (based on DM1000 [46]) is added to the system. The rangefinders are connected to the sensor nodes on the feet. To obtain the best performance of the distance measurement, the two rangefinders are placed at the medial side of foot, close to the heel, antennas face to face, as shown in **Figure 12**. The feet relative distance provided by the modules is coupled with the information from sensors on the feet to determine the IC and EC events and the times they occur. The rangefinders are sampled at 100 Hz. **Figure 3** illustrates the main organization and role of the elements of the final system.

4.3 Experiments

Experiments are conducted to evaluate the accuracy of the proposed system including the gait event detection and joint angle estimation. Experiments are performed in a gait analysis laboratory equipped with 3D-GA system. Totally, 11 hemiparetic patients, 4 females and 7 males 51.7 ± 18.2 years old, participated in the experiments. About, 4 healthy people, 1 female and 3 male aged 24 ± 3.1 years, participated in the experiments. The persons were equipped with both markers for 3D-GA system and proposed wearable system during experiment. All persons have been asked to walk 6 times on a straight course of 8 m with self-selected confirmable speed. The walking scenarios are captured by 3D-GA system at 100 Hz and at 70 Hz by the proposed wearable system. The embedded system's records are re-sampled at 100 Hz so that they can be compared point-to-point with those of the 3D-GA system.

Figure 13 illustrates the joint angles of a hemiparetic patient normalized in gait cycles. In this figure, the red curves represent the joint angles of the left side (healthy side) and the blue curves represent the joint angles of the right side (paretic side). The dotted curves are the angles measured by the 3D-GA system and the solid lines are the angles estimated by the proposed wearable system.

The two systems are compared by evaluating the accuracy of the gait event detection (IC and FC) and the joint angle estimation. IC and FC events' RSMEs are used to evaluate the accuracy of gait event detection, and the detection rate is calculated to describe the robustness of event detection.

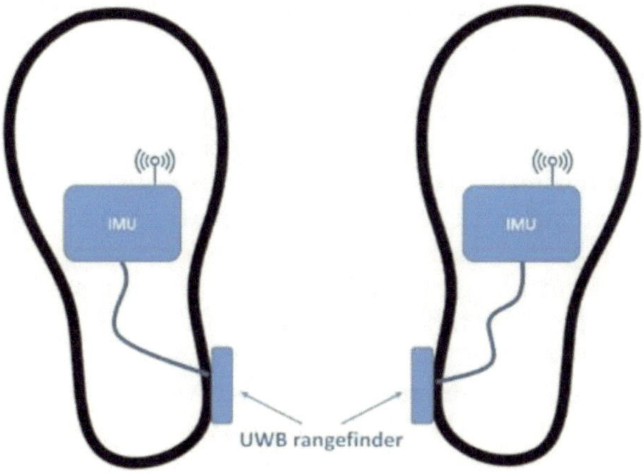

Figure 12.
Placement of rangefinder.

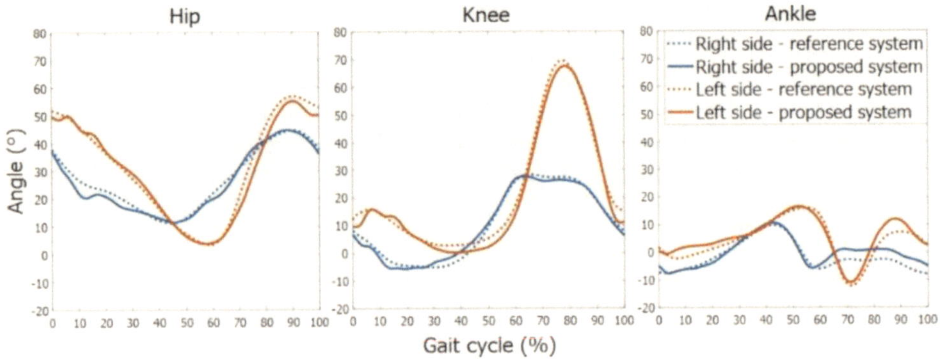

Figure 13.
Joint angles of hemiparetic subject normalized in gait cycle.

Table 2 summarizes the results of the comparison of the accuracy between the proposed system and the 3D-GA system of joint angles and gait events as well as the robustness of the gait event detection. The RMSE estimates of joint angles are between 1.3° and 3.9° for hemiparetic patients and between 1.8° and 4° for healthy subjects. The CCs for stroke subjects are between 0.9 and 0.99. For healthy persons, they are between 0.91 and 0.99. In terms of the detection of gait events, the RSMEs for IC detection are between 45 and 14 ms for hemiparetic patients and between 16 and 24 ms for healthy persons. The FC event detection has a precision between 12 and 41 ms for hemiparetic patients and between 15 and 20 ms for healthy persons. The rates of detection of CI are between 93 and 100% for hemiparetic patients and between 95 and 100% for healthy persons. The rates of detection of FC are between 92 and 100% for hemiparetic patients and between 97 and 100% for healthy people.

Figure 14 illustrates the correlation and concordance of the joint angles measured by the two systems. The coefficient of determination (r^2) equals 0.98. The lower limits of agreement (95%) equal −3.6° and the upper limits of agreement (95%) equal 5.9°.

4.4 Discussion

This chapter describes the use of a wireless rangefinder to measure the feet relative distance in order to automatically detect the gait events (IC and FC) in everyday life condition and specially to consider the differences between normal and pathological walking.

To evaluate the precision and robustness of the proposed system, experiments have been carried out on hemiparetic and healthy persons. The estimated information delivered is compared with that from the 3D-GA system. Their comparison shows that the joint angles estimated with the proposed system are quite comparable to those of the reference system. In terms of the detection of gait events, thanks to the additional information given by the rangefinders, errors are rare. The system is very robust in the case of pathological walking.

In terms of detection of gait events, the results show a precision of 27 ms for IC events of hemiparetic patients and 22 ms for FC events. More than 98% of the events are correctly detected. The results show that this method has good accuracy and is especially robust for pathological gait. However, because of the limitation of the area detectable by the 3D-GA system, the comparison can be done only between the data captured in this area. So, even if the detection rate of the events of several persons reaches 100%, one can imagine that it is possible that some events are lost during the beginning and the end of the gait.

		Joint angles						Gait events			
		Ankle		Knee		Hip		CI		CF	
		RMSE (°)	CC	RMSE (°)	CC	RMSE (°)	CC	RMSE (ms)	Rate (%)	RMSE (ms)	Rate (%)
Hemiparetic patients	1	2.1	0.95	1.9	0.99	2.3	0.98	43	100	17	100
	2	3.9	0.92	1.9	0.98	3.8	0.98	22	100	22	97
	3	2.4	0.97	2.6	0.99	3.8	0.94	25	97	17	100
	4	1.8	0.92	3.9	0.98	3.9	0.92	20	100	22	100
	5	2.6	0.94	2.9	0.99	2.6	0.98	45	98	42	98
	6	2.6	0.91	2.5	0.99	2.7	0.98	15	100	13	100
	7	3.9	0.95	3.5	0.98	3.5	0.97	35	100	41	100
	8	3.6	0.90	2.4	0.99	3	0.99	19	100	12	100
	9	2.9	0.93	3.1	0.97	3.6	0.91	28	98	15	97
	10	1.9	0.97	1.8	0.99	1.6	0.99	14	100	17	100
	11	2.5	0.95	1.3	0.99	3.6	0.99	30	93	24	92
Mean		2.75	0.94	2.53	0.99	3.13	0.97	26.91	98.73	22.00	98.55
Healthy persons	1	3.2	0.92	1.9	0.99	3.3	0.97	20	97	15	100
	2	3.1	0.94	3.7	0.98	1.2	0.99	24	98	13	97
	3	4	0.91	1.8	0.99	1.5	0.99	21	95	20	97
	4	2.7	0.93	3	0.99	2.8	0.98	16	100	12	100
Mean		3.25	0.93	2.60	0.99	2.20	0.98	20.25	97.50	15.00	98.50

Table 2.
Comparison between the proposed system and the 3D-GA system.

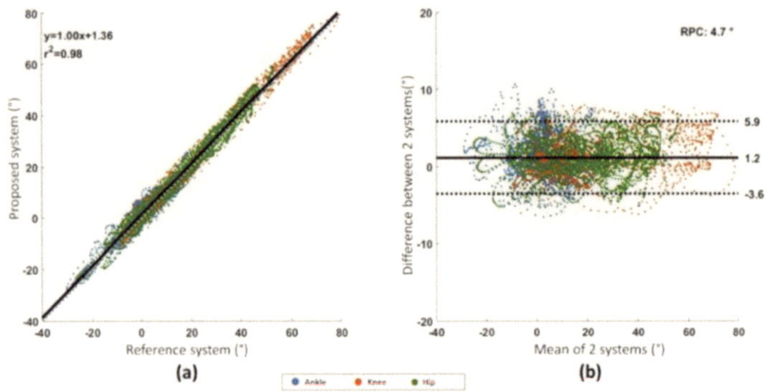

Figure 14.
Correlation (a) and Bland-Altman plot (b).

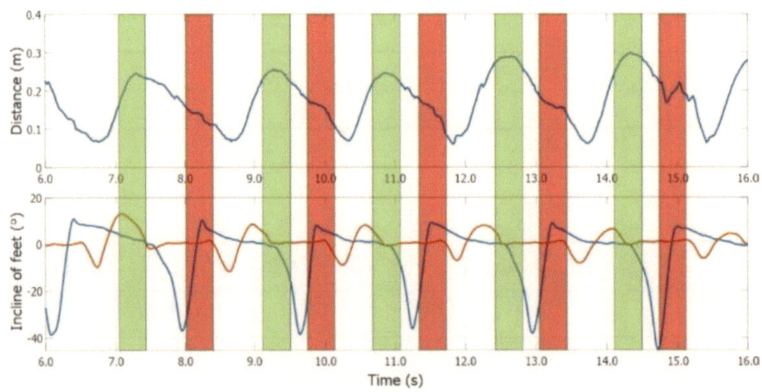

Figure 15.
CI nondetectable case.

The proposed system provides good accuracy in determining hemiparetic events but has a limitation. The method uses the relative distance between the feet as the main source of information to determine the IC event. Then, the FC is searched between two IC events. As a result, if the IC event is not correctly determined, the FC event cannot be detected. As shown in **Figure 11**, the IC events of both feet correspond to the local maximum of the relative distance signal of the feet. If the peaks corresponding to the IC are very attenuated, the risk of no longer detecting the IC event increases (**Figure 15**). This figure shows the relative distance and inclinations of the two feet. The colored areas represent the areas where the peaks on the distance signal corresponding to the IC must be observed. In green zones, significant peaks are observable; in red zones, most peaks are very attenuated or undetectable. This system cannot then be used on people that walk with a maximum distance of the feet very close to the length of the step during the double phase support. In practice, for all persons that have a minimum relative distance between feet larger than 20 cm, this system works properly.

5. Conclusion and perspectives

The chapter describes a wireless embedded system used to record information related to the gait of patients with after-effects of stroke in ecological situations.

It is based on the use of seven inertial sensors. Each sensor executes the orientation estimation algorithm. Even if each sensor uses its local clock and performs the measurement according to its own time base, their synchronization through reference broadcast time synchronization (RBTS) allows synchronization accuracy, synchronization speed, and the number of sensors to synchronize. Other constraints related to the use of the wireless link are the speed of transmission and energy consumption. To address these constraints, among wireless transmission technologies, we selected a proprietary protocol that allows the clock error between two sensors limited to a value less than 37.6 μs that does not accumulate over time. Thanks to the efficiency of this protocol, the sampling frequency to transmit the raw measurements and the orientation of the segments estimated by the sensors reaches 109 Hz.

The embedded wireless system uses a pair of range-finders to determine the gait events to split the recordings into gait cycles and calculate the temporal parameters. The method to determine the gait events, initial contact (IC) and final contact (FC), uses relative distance between feet and speed angular feet. The system also estimates the articular angles of the lower limbs. This information is the input of a piece of post-processing software that determines the temporal parameters and automatically cuts the joint angles into walking cycles. A series of experiments was conducted to evaluate the accuracy and robustness of the system. The difference between the values measured by the embedded system and the 3D-GA system shows a good robustness on the pathological path, which is quite innovative.

This development shows the evolution of our embedded gait analysis system. The final system provides the measured quantities comparable to those from a 3D-GA system. The algorithmic and material design takes into account the constraints of pathological walking and use in an ecological situation. The algorithms for segment orientation estimation and gait event detection are optimized for pathological walking. The new method we have proposed for determining the events of walking improves the robustness of event detection in the pathological case. In order for the system to be used in an ecological situation and to record the activity of the person in his daily life, the electronic design of the system is carried out in order to minimize the influence of the system on the walking of people and to have enough autonomy to record walking all day long. An effort has also been made to improve the ease of implementation and use.

In addition, it is possible to analyze the walk in more complex or functional situations. Indeed, certain clinical tests required different movements on the patient. This is the case, for example, for the TUG (Timed Up and Go). This test requires the patient to get up from a chair, walk forward 3 m, turn around a pad, walk back, and then sit down again. This test involves several motor skills. According to the chronometric performance, the risk of falling for the patient was identified for a number of values. We also looked to turn strategies in this test for stroke patients compared to healthy subjects from the quantification of the pelvis trajectory [47]. To make these comparisons, DTW (Dynamic Time Warping) methods on the trajectory of the basin on the horizontal plane were used. These methods allow identification of patients' strategies and therefore their classification as shown in [48, 49]. It is realistic to hypothesize on walking route (straight lines, stairs, up and down slopes, etc.), identification of displacement strategies from the calculation of the DTW on joint kinematics and/or segmental accelerations to follow the evolution (improvement or degradation) of the locomotor possibilities of the patient. This promising approach is the main line of our current work.

Author details

Gilbert Pradel[1*], Tong Li[1], Didier Pradon[2] and Nicolas Roche[1,2]

1 END-ICAP Lab. - UMR 1179, French National Institute for Health and Medical Research, Montigny-le-Bretonneux, France

2 Raymond Poincaré Teaching Hospital (APHP), Garches, France

*Address all correspondence to: gilbert.pradel@ens-paris-saclay.fr

References

[1] Öken Ö, Yavuzer G, Ergöçen S, Yorgancıoglu ZR, Stam HJ. Repeatability and variation of quantitative gait data in subgroups of patients with stroke. Gait & Posture. 2008;**27**(3):506-511

[2] Mazzaro N, Nielsen JF, Grey MJ, Sinkjaer T. Decreased contribution from afferent feedback to the soleus muscle during walking in patients with spastic stroke. Journal of Stroke and Cerebrovascular Diseases. 2007;**16**(4):135-144

[3] Perry J, Burnfield JM. Gait Analysis: Normal and Pathological Function. 2nd ed. Thorofare, NJ: SLACK; 2010. 551 p

[4] Williams PE, Goldspink G. Changes in sarcomere length and physiological properties in immobilized muscle. Journal of Anatomy. 1978;**127**(Pt 3):459-468

[5] Bohannon RW, Andrews AW, Smith MB. Rehabilitation goals of patients with hemiplegia. International Journal of Rehabilitation Research. 1988;**11**(2):181-184

[6] Mumma CM. Perceived losses following stroke. Rehabilitation Nursing. 2000;**25**(5):192-195

[7] Pound P, Gompertz P, Ebrahim S. A patient-centred study of the consequences of stroke. Clinical Rehabilitation. 1998;**12**(4):338-347

[8] Ng SS, Tsang WW, Cheung TH, Chung JS, To FP, Yu PC. Walkway length, but not turning direction, determines the six-minute walk test distance in individuals with stroke. Archives of Physical Medicine and Rehabilitation. 2011;**92**(5):806-811

[9] Beekman E, Mesters I, Hendriks EJM, Klaassen MPM, Gosselink R, van Schayck OCP, et al. Course length of 30 metres versus 10 metres has a significant influence on six-minute walk distance in patients with COPD: An experimental crossover study. Journal of Physiotherapy. 2013;**59**(3):169-176

[10] Kharb A, Saini V, Jain YK, Dhiman S. A review of gait cycle and its parameters. International Journal of Computational Engineering & Management. 2011;**13**:6

[11] Whittle MW. Clinical gait analysis: A review. Human Movement Science. 1996;**15**(3):369-387

[12] Brandstater ME, de Bruin H, Gowland C, Clark BM. Hemiplegic gait: Analysis of temporal variables. Archives of Physical Medicine and Rehabilitation. 1983;**64**(12):583-587

[13] Knutsson E, Richards C. Different types of disturbed motor control in gait of hemiparetic patients. Brain: A Journal of Neurology. 1979;**102**(2):405-430

[14] Olney SJ, Griffin MP, McBride ID, et al. Temporal, kinematic, and kinetic variables related to gait speed in subjects with hemiplegia: A regression approach. Physical Therapy. 1994;**74**(9):872

[15] Turnbull GI, Charteris J, Wall JC. A comparison of the range of walking speeds between normal and hemiplegic subjects. Scandinavian Journal of Rehabilitation Medicine. 1995;**27**(3):175-182

[16] Hsu A-L, Tang P-F, Jan M-H. Analysis of impairments influencing gait velocity and asymmetry of hemiplegic patients after mild to moderate stroke1. Archives of Physical Medicine and Rehabilitation. 2003;**84**(8):1185-1193

[17] Woolley SM. Characteristics of gait in hemiplegia. Topics in Stroke Rehabilitation. 2001;**7**(4):1-18

[18] Balaban B, Tok F. Gait disturbances in patients with stroke. PM&R. 2014;**6**(7):635-642

[19] Olney SJ, Richards C. Hemiparetic gait following stroke. Part I: Characteristics. Gait & Posture. 1996;**4**(2):136-148

[20] Olney SJ, Griffin MP, Monga TN, McBride ID. Work and power in gait of stroke patients. Archives of Physical Medicine and Rehabilitation. 1991;**72**(5):309-314

[21] Berger W, Horstmann G, Dietz V. Tension development and muscle activation in the leg during gait in spastic hemiparesis: Independence of muscle hypertonia and exaggerated stretch reflexes. Journal of Neurology, Neurosurgery, and Psychiatry. 1984;**47**(9):1029-1033

[22] Dietz V, Sinkjaer T. Spastic movement disorder: Impaired reflex function and altered muscle mechanics. Lancet Neurology. 2007;**6**(8):725-733

[23] Zhou H, Nicholls C, Kunz T, Schwartz H. Frequency accuracy & stability dependencies of crystal oscillators. Carlet Univ Syst Comput Eng Tech Rep SCE-08-12 [Internet]. 2008. Available from: http://kunz-pc.sce.carleton.ca/thesis/CrystalOscillators.pdf

[24] Shuster MD. Survey of attitude representations. The Journal of the Astronautical Sciences. 1993;**41**:439-517

[25] Phillips WF, Hailey CE, Gebert GA. Review of attitude representations used for aircraft kinematics. Journal of Aircraft. 2001;**38**(4):718-737

[26] Li T, Pradel G. Embedded gait parameter acquisition system for hemiplegic persons—HemiGaitEm. In: Mechatronics, Mechatronics Forum International Conference, 14. Karlstad: Karlstad University; 2014. pp. 1-8

[27] Madgwick SOH, Harrison AJL, Vaidyanathan R. Estimation of IMU and MARG orientation using a gradient descent algorithm. In: 2011 IEEE International Conference on Rehabilitation Robotics. 2011. pp. 1-7

[28] Schwartz MH, Trost JP, Wervey RA. Measurement and management of errors in quantitative gait data. Gait & Posture. 2004;**20**(2):196-203

[29] Seel T, Raisch J, Schauer T. IMU-based joint angle measurement for gait analysis. Sensors. 2014;**14**(4):6891-6909

[30] Aminian K, Najafi B, Büla C, Leyvraz P-F, Robert P. Spatio-temporal parameters of gait measured by an ambulatory system using miniature gyroscopes. Journal of Biomechanics. 2002;**35**(5):689-699

[31] Micó-Amigo ME, Kingma I, Ainsworth E, Walgaard S, Niessen M, van Lummel RC, et al. A novel accelerometry-based algorithm for the detection of step durations over short episodes of gait in healthy elderly. Journal of NeuroEngineering and Rehabilitation. 2016;**13**(1). Available from: http://jneuroengrehab.biomedcentral.com/articles/10.1186/s12984-016-0145-6

[32] Pappas IP, Popovic MR, Keller T, Dietz V, Morari M. A reliable gait phase detection system. IEEE Transactions on Neural Systems and Rehabilitation Engineering. 2001;**9**(2):113-125

[33] Pappas IPI, Keller T, Mangold S, Popovic MR, Dietz V, Morari M. A reliable gyroscope-based gait-phase detection sensor embedded in a shoe insole. IEEE Sensors Journal. 2004;**4**(2):268-274

[34] Kotiadis D, Hermens HJ, Veltink PH. Inertial gait phase detection for control of a drop foot stimulator: Inertial sensing for gait phase detection. Medical Engineering & Physics. 2010;**32**(4):287-297

[35] Mansfield A, Lyons GM. The use of accelerometry to detect heel contact events for use as a sensor in FES assisted

walking. Medical Engineering & Physics. 2003;**25**(10):879-885

[36] Trojaniello D, Cereatti A, Pelosin E, Avanzino L, Mirelman A, Hausdorff JM, et al. Estimation of step-by-step spatio-temporal parameters of normal and impaired gait using shank-mounted magneto-inertial sensors: Application to elderly, hemiparetic, parkinsonian and choreic gait. Journal of NeuroEngineering and Rehabilitation. 2014;**11**:152

[37] Rueterbories J, Spaich EG, Larsen B, Andersen OK. Methods for gait event detection and analysis in ambulatory systems. Medical Engineering & Physics. 2010;**32**(6):545-552

[38] Sabatini AM, Martelloni C, Scapellato S, Cavallo F. Assessment of walking features from foot inertial sensing. IEEE Transactions on Biomedical Engineering. 2005;**52**(3):486-494

[39] Gouwanda D, Gopalai AA. A robust real-time gait event detection using wireless gyroscope and its application on normal and altered gaits. Medical Engineering & Physics. 2015;**37**(2):219-225

[40] Jimenez AR, Seco F, Prieto JC, Guevara J. Indoor pedestrian navigation using an INS/EKF framework for yaw drift reduction and a foot-mounted IMU. In IEEE; 2010. pp. 135-143. Available from: http://ieeexplore.ieee.org/document/5649300/

[41] Ojeda L, Borenstein J. Non-GPS navigation for security personnel and first responders. Journal of Navigation. 2007;**60**(03):391-407

[42] Bebek Ö, Suster MA, Rajgopal S, Fu MJ, Huang X, Çavusoglu MC, et al. Personal navigation via high-resolution gait-corrected inertial measurement units. IEEE Transactions on Instrumentation and Measurement. 2010;**59**(11):3018-3027

[43] Wang Z, Zhao H, Qiu S, Gao Q. Stance-phase detection for ZUPT-aided foot-mounted pedestrian navigation system. IEEE/ASME Transactions on Mechatronics. 2015;**20**(6):3170-3181

[44] Nilsson J-O, Skog I, Händel P. A note on the limitations of ZUPTs and the implications on sensor error modeling. In: 2012 International Conference on Indoor Positioning and Indoor Navigation (IPIN), 13-15th November 2012. 2012. Available from: http://www.diva-portal.org/smash/record.jsf?pid=diva2:575831

[45] Skog I, Nilsson J-O, Handel P. Evaluation of zero-velocity detectors for foot-mounted inertial navigation systems. Proc IPIN [Internet]. 2010. Available from: http://ieeexplore.ieee.org/xpls/abs_all.jsp?arnumber=5646936

[46] DW1000 Radio IC [Internet]. Decawave. 2018. Available from: https://www.decawave.com/product/dw1000-radio-ic/

[47] Bonnyaud C, Roche N, Van Hamme A, Bensmail D, Pradon D. Locomotor trajectories of stroke patients during oriented gait and turning. PLoS ONE. 2016;**11**(2). Available from: https://www.ncbi.nlm.nih.gov/pmc/articles/PMC4760702/

[48] Rybarczyk Y, Deters JK, Gonzalo AA, Esparza D, Gonzalez M, Villarreal S, et al. Recognition of physiotherapeutic exercises through DTW and low-cost vision-based motion capture. In: Nunes IL, editor. Advances in Human Factors and Systems Interaction (Advances in Intelligent Systems and Computing). Springer International Publishing; 2018. pp. 348-360

[49] Rybarczyk Y, Leconte L, Medina JP. Telerehabilitation Platform for Post-Arthroplasty Recovery: A Dynamic Time Warping Approach. p. 6

Chapter 9

Improvement of Cooperative Action for Multi-Agent System by Rewards Distribution

Mengchun Xie

Abstract

The frequency of natural disasters is increasing everywhere in the world, which is a major impediment to sustainable development. One important issue for the international community is to reduce vulnerability to and damage from disasters. In addition, a large number of injuries occur simultaneously in a large-scale disaster, and the condition of the injured will change over time. Efficient rescue activities are carried out using triage to determine the priority of injury treatment based on the severity of the persons' conditions. In this chapter, we discuss acquiring cooperative behavior of rescuing the injured and clearing obstacles according to triage of the injured in a multi-agent system. We propose three methods of reward distribution: (1) reward distribution responding to the condition of the injured, (2) reward distribution based on the contribution degree, and (3) reward distribution by the contribution degree responding to the condition of the injured. We investigated the effectiveness of the three proposed methods for a disaster relief problem by an experiment. The results of the experiment showed that agents gained high rewards by rescuing those in most urgent need under the method having the reward distributed according to the contribution degree responding to the condition of the injured.

Keywords: multi-agent system, reinforcement learning, reward distribution, triage, disaster relief problem

1. Introduction

The frequency of natural disasters is increasing everywhere in the world, which is a major impediment to sustainable development. In order to minimize the damage of disasters, the United Nations Office for Disaster Risk Reduction (UNISDR) calls for the promotion of disaster prevention and mitigation by local governments in each country. This is an important issue for the international community in order to reduce vulnerability to and damage from disasters.

In the case of a large-scale disaster, a large number of injuries occur simultaneously, and the condition of the injured changes with the lapse of time. This implies that, to conduct efficient treatment when resources are insufficient to immediately treat all the people who are injured, it is necessary to use triage, which is the process of determining the priority of treatment based on the severity of the injured person's condition [1].

To date, many different remote-controlled disaster relief robots have been developed. A further complication, besides the need for triage, is that these robots must work in environments in which communication is not always secure. For these reasons, there is a need for autonomous disaster relief robots, that is, robots which can learn from the conditions that they encounter and then take independent action [2]. Thus, efficient rescue needs to consider the condition of the injured, which changes with the lapse of time, even with the use of disaster rescue robots.

Reinforcement learning is one way that robots can acquire information about appropriate behavior in new environments. Under this learning system, robots can observe the environment, select and perform actions, and obtain rewards [3–6]. Each robot must learn what the best policy (i.e., the policy that obtains the largest amount of reward over time) is by itself.

Recent research on disaster relief robots has included consideration of multi-agent systems, that is, systems that include two or more disaster relief robots. A multi-agent system in which multiple agents explore sections of damaged building with the goal of updating a topological map of the building with safe routes is discussed [7, 8]. John et al. constructed a multi-agent systems approach to disaster situation management, which is a complex multidimensional process involving a large number of mobile interoperating agents [9]. However, to successfully interact in the real world, agents must be able to reason about their interactions with heterogeneous agents of widely varying properties and capabilities. It is necessary that agents are able to learn from the environment and implement independent actions by using perceptual and reasoning in order to carry out their task in the best possible way [10, 11].

Numerous studies regarding learning in multi-agent systems have been conducted. Spychalski and Arendt proposed a methodology for implementing machine learning capability in multi-agent systems for aided design of selected control systems allowed to improve their performance by reducing the time spent processing requests that were previously acknowledged and stored in the learning module [12]. In [13], a new kind of multi-agent reinforcement learning algorithm, called TM_Qlearning, which combines traditional Q-learning with observation-based teammate modeling techniques, was proposed. Two multi-agent reinforcement learning methods, both consisting of promoting the selection of actions so that the chosen action not only relies on the present experience but also on an estimation of possible future ones, have been proposed to better solve the coordination problem and the exploration/exploitation dilemma in the case of nonstationary environments [14]. In [15], the construction of a multi-agent evacuation guidance simulation that consists of evacuee agents and instruction agents was reported, and the optimum evacuation guidance method was discussed through numerical simulations by using the multi-agent system for post-earthquake tsunami events. A simulation of a disaster relief problem that included multiple autonomous robots working as a multi-agent system has been reported [16].

In disaster relief problems, it is important to rescue the injured and remove obstacles according to conditions that are changing with the passage of time. However, conventional research on multiple agents targeted for disaster relief has not taken into consideration the condition of the injured, so it is insufficient for efficient rescue.

In this chapter, we discuss acquiring cooperative behavior of rescuing the injured and clearing obstacles according to triage of the injured in a multi-agent system. We propose three methods of reward distribution: (1) reward distribution responding to the condition of the injured, (2) reward distribution based on the contribution degree, and (3) reward distribution by the contribution degree responding to the condition of the injured. We investigated the effectiveness of these proposed methods for a disaster relief problem by an experiment. The results of the experiment showed that agents gained high rewards by rescuing those in most urgent need under the method having the reward distributed according to the contribution degree responding to the condition of the injured.

2. Learning of multi-agent systems and representation of disaster relief problem

2.1 Learning of multi-agent systems

Agents are a computational mechanism that exist in some complex environment, sense and perform actions in its environment, and by doing so realize a set of tasks for which it is assigned. A multi-agent system consists of agents that interact with each other, situated in a common environment, which they perceive with sensors and upon which they act with actuators (**Figure 1**). Agent and environment are relationships of the interaction. In the meantime, when the environments are inaccessible, the information which can be perceived from the environment is limited, and it is inaccurate, and it entails delay [2, 17, 18].

In [19], the following major characteristics of multi-agent systems were identified:

- Each agent has incomplete information and is restricted in its capabilities.
- The control of the system is distributed.
- The data are decentralized.
- The computation is asynchronous.

In multi-agent systems, individual agents are forced to engage with other agents that have varying goals, abilities, and composition. Reinforcement learning have been used to learn about other agents and adapt local behavior for the purpose of achieving coordination in multi-agent situations in which the individual agents are not aware of each another [20].

Various reinforcement learning strategies have been proposed that can be used by agents to develop a policy to maximizing rewards accumulated over time. A prominent algorithm in reinforcement learning is the Q-learning algorithm.

In Q-learning, the decision policy is represented by the Q-factors, which estimates long-term discounted rewards for each state-action pair. Let $Q(s, a)$ denote the

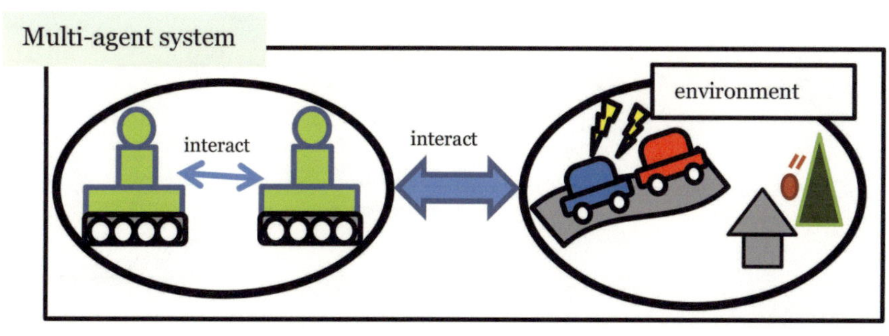

Figure 1.
Multi-agent systems.

Q-factor for state s and action a. If an action a in state s produces a reinforcement of r and a transition to state s_{t+1}, then the corresponding Q-factor is modified as follows:

$$Q(s_t, a_t) \leftarrow Q(s_t, a_t) + \alpha[r + \gamma max Q(s_{t+1}, a) - Q(S_t, a_t)] \quad (1)$$

where α is a small constant called learning rate, which denotes a step-size parameter in the iteration, and γ denotes the discounting factor. Theoretically, the algorithm is allowed to run for infinitely many iterations until the Q-factors converge.

2.2 The target problem

In this chapter, we focus on a disaster relief as a target problem similar to previous research [16]. In the disaster relief problem, agents must rescue the injured as quickly as possible, and the injured with different severity and urgency of the condition are placed on a field of fixed size. Because there are multiple injured and obstacles, the disaster relief problem can be considered to be a multi-agent system. Each agent focuses on achieving its own target, and the task of system is to efficiently rescue all of the injured and remove obstacles (**Figure 2**).

Efficient rescue is performed at a disaster site using triage to assign priority of transport or treatment based on the severity and urgency of the condition of the injured. In the disaster rescue problem, it is thus necessary to reflect triage based on the condition of the injured. For this purpose, in this chapter, we designate the condition of the injured as red (requiring emergency treatment), yellow (requiring urgent treatment), green (light injury), or black (lifesaving is difficult) in descending order of urgency.

The disaster relief problem is represented as shown in **Figure 3**. The field is divided into an N × N lattice. Agents are indicated by circles, ◎; the injured are indicated by R, Y, G, and B; removable obstacles are indicated by white triangles, △; and nonremovable obstacles are indicated by black triangles, ▲. The destination of injures is indicated by a white square, □; and the collection site of movable obstacles is indicated by a black square, ■. A single step is defined such that each of the agents on the field completes a single action, and the field is re-initialized once all of the injured have been moved.

The agents considered in this chapter are depicted in **Figure 4** and included two types, to obtain cooperative actions. The rescue agents have the primary function of rescuing the injured, and the removal agents have the primary function of removing obstacles, although either type can perform both functions. The agents

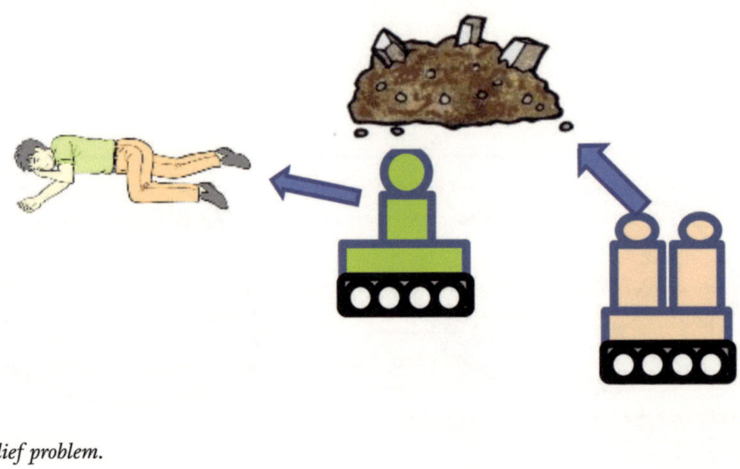

Figure 2.
Disaster relief problem.

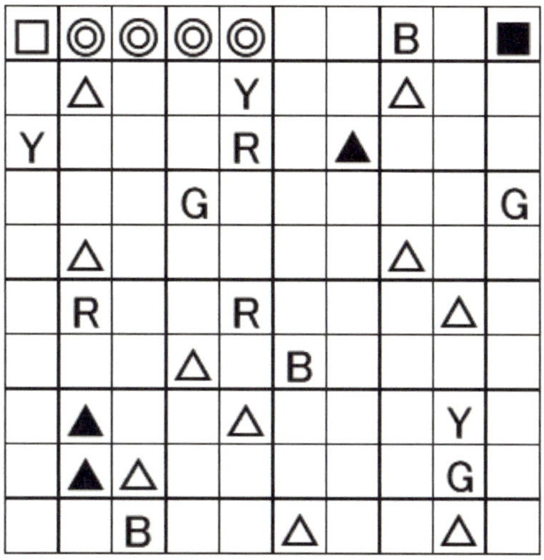

Figure 3.
An example of representation for a disaster relief problem.

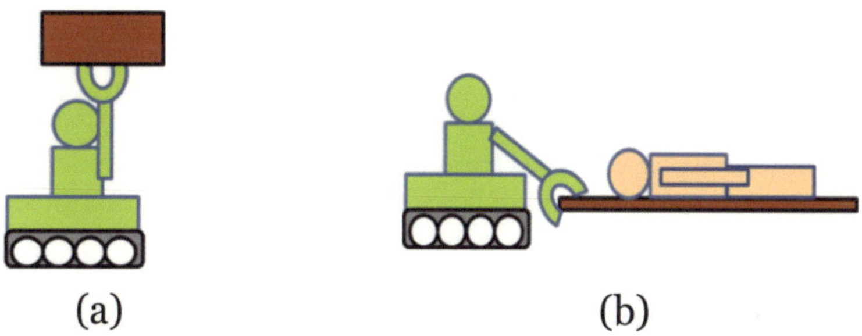

Figure 4.
Agents of different functions: (a) removing agent and (b) relief agent.

recognize the colors of the injured on the field and identify the condition of the injured in correspondence with those colors.

Each agent considers the overall tasks in the given environment, carries out the tasks in accordance with the assigned roles, and learns appropriate actions that bring high rewards.

An agent can recognize its circumstance within a prescribed field of vision and move one cell vertically or horizontally, but will stay in place without moving if a nonremovable obstacle, injured transport destination, obstacle transport destination, or other agent occupies the movement destination or if the movement destination is outside the field. Each agent has a constant but limited view of the field, and it can assess the surrounding environment.

The available actions of agents are (1) moving up, down, right, or left to an adjacent cell; (2) remaining in the present cell when adjacent cell is occupied by an obstacle that cannot be removed or by another agent; and (3) finding an injured person or a movable obstacle and taking it to the appropriate location.

If an agent is processing an injured person and next action is moving it to the appropriate destination, then the task of the agent is completed. The agent can begin a new task for rescuing or removing. When all of the injured on the field have been rescued, the overall task is completed.

3. Improvement of Cooperative Action by Rewards Distribution

3.1 Cooperative agents

In multi-agent system, the environment changes from static to dynamic because multiple autonomous agents exist. An agent engaged in cooperative action decides its actions by referring to not only its own information and purpose but to those of other agents as well [16]. The cooperative agents are acquired by sharing sensation, sharing episodes, and sharing learned policies [17, 19–21]. Cooperative actions are important not only in situations where multiple agents have to work together to accomplish a common goal but also in situations where each agents has its own goal [22].

In this chapter, the multi-agent systems are composed of agents' different behaviors. One is to perform relief (*relief agents*), and the other is to remove obstacles (*removing agents*). Cooperation was achieved by giving different rewards to different behaviors.

3.2 Reward distribution with consideration of condition of the injured

It is necessary to have the multi-agent systems learn efficient rescue with the condition of the injured taken into consideration.

Prior studies used reward distribution with the reward value differing in accordance with the agent action but gave no consideration to the condition of the injured.

In this chapter, we propose three types of reward distribution as methods for obtaining cooperative action of injured rescue and obstacle removal in accordance with the urgency of the condition of the injured.

3.2.1 Method 1: reward distribution responding to the condition of the injured

A conferred reward is high in value when an injured person in a condition of high urgency is rescued and decreases in value for those in less urgent conditions. Thus, $R_r > R_y > R_g > R_b$, where R_r, R_y, R_g, and R_b are the reward values for the rescue of injured persons in the red, yellow, green, and black condition categories, respectively.

3.2.2 Method 2: reward distribution based on the contribution degree

In Method 2, the reward value reflects the time spent by the rescue agent as the contribution degree.

With R as the basic reward value when the rescue agent completes the injured rescue, C as the contribution degree, and λ as a weighting factor, the reward r earned by the rescue agent in learning is as given by Eq. (2). A large λ results in a reward that is greatly augmented relative to the basic reward, according to contribution degree.

Assessed contribution degree C increases with decreasing time spent in rescuing the injured, as shown in Eq. (3), in which T_e is the time of completion of rescue of all the injured by the rescue agents and T_i is the time spent by an agent to rescue an injured person.

$$r = (1 + \lambda C)R \tag{2}$$

$$C = T_i / T_e \tag{3}$$

3.2.3 Method 3: reward distribution by the contribution degree responding to the condition of the injured

In Eq. (2), basic reward value R at the time of completion of each task takes on one of the values $R_r > R_y > R_g > R_b$ according to the condition of the injured person.

4. Experimental results and discussion

4.1 Experimental conditions

In the study presented in this chapter, we experimented on obtaining cooperative action by agents for efficient rescue in accordance with the condition of the injured and obstacle removal, using the three proposed reward distributions. We assigned the injured and obstacle transport destinations to one cell each on the field shown in **Figure 3** and numbers of agents, injured persons, and obstacles as listed in **Table 1**. The mean of five simulation trials was taken as the result.

4.2 Effects of reward distribution timing

We investigated the effects of the three patterns of reward distribution timing on task completion on the efficiency of learning injured rescue. The reward is given when an injured person or obstacle is discovered in Pattern 1. The reward is given when an injured person or object is taken for removal to the appropriate location in Pattern 2. Rewards are given twice in Pattern 3: at the stage of discovering an injured person or obstacle and at the stage where transportation is completed.

The results of an experiment to compare the three reward distribution timing patterns are shown in **Figure 5**. The horizontal axis represents the episodes, and the vertical axis represents the number of steps for task completion by all agents. These results indicate that Pattern 3 allowed completion of the tasks in a smaller number

The setting of field		
The field size		10 × 10
The number of rescue agents		2
The number of clearing agents		2
The number of injured individuals	Red	3
	Yellow	3
	Green	3
	Black	3
The number of removal of possible obstacles		10
The number of removal of impossible obstacles		3
The setting of agent		
Learning rate α		0.1
Discount rate γ		0.9
Greedy policy ε		0.1

Table 1.
Experimental conditions.

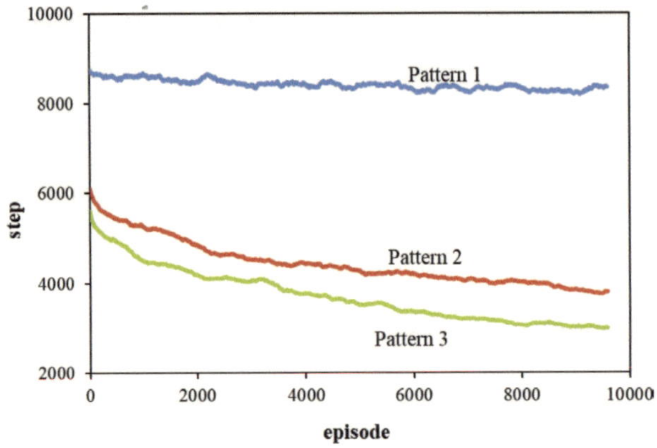

Figure 5.
Results of experiment to compare three reward distribution timing patterns.

of steps than did Patterns 1 and 2, which in turn indicates that efficient rescue and removal was learned by conferring rewards in two stages and thus led the agent to regard the course from discovery to transport as one task. We therefore applied Pattern 3 in the subsequent experiments.

4.3 Obtaining cooperative action that considers the condition of the injured and the effects of reward distribution timing

We applied the three types of reward distributions in experiments for efficient rescue in accordance with the urgency of the condition of the injured. In the following descriptions of experimental results, the horizontal axis represents episodes, and the vertical axis represents the number of steps for task completion by all agents.

Figure 6 shows the results of an experiment to investigate the effectiveness of a reward distribution in accordance with condition (Method 1) compared to the conventional method [16]. As shown, the number of steps is higher throughout with Method 1 than with the standard method, thus indicating learning to postpone rescue of the low urgency injured and prioritize rescue of the high urgency injured.

Finally, we performed an experiment to investigate the effectiveness of reward distribution based on contribution degree (Method 2) in comparison to Method 1 and another experiment to investigate the effectiveness of reward distribution by contribution degree in accordance with injured condition (Method 3) in

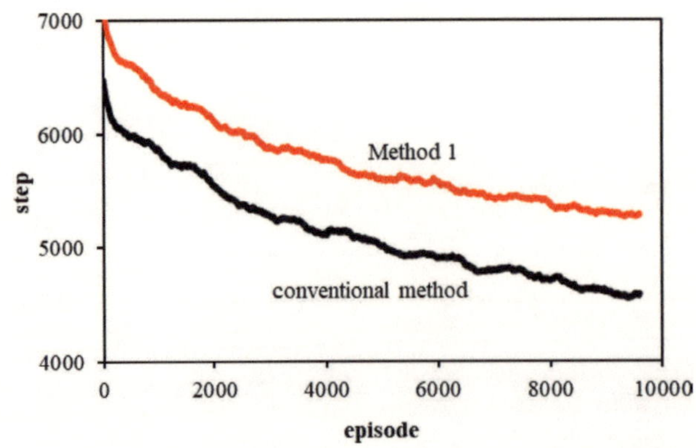

Figure 6.
Results of the conventional method and proposed Method 1.

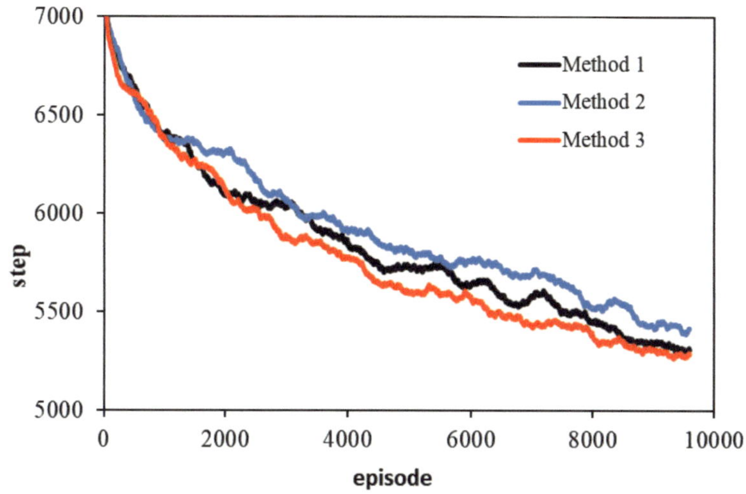

Figure 7.
Results of the different proposed methods.

Triage of injured	Method 1	Method 2	Method 3
Red	1126.73	1140.93	1102.93
Yellow	1518.20	1614.40	1269.07
Green	2404.53	2499.33	1685.47
Black	3284.27	2999.47	2447.33

Table 2.
Mean step numbers by different reward distribution.

comparison with the other proposed methods (Methods 1 and 2). The results are shown in **Figure 7** and **Table 2**.

As shown, Method 2 tends to yield a higher number of steps than Method 1 in and after around episode 6000. This indicates that, for efficient injured rescue with consideration for contribution degree, the rescue order learned was to first rescue those injured who were nearby and thus shorten the rescue time, leaving for later the rescue of those who were farther away.

Method 3 is approximately 2.2 and 3.4% superior to Methods 1 and 2, respectively. The agents were apparently able to learn rescue of the injured in accordance with urgency because a reward differing in accordance with injured condition was conferred on the agents. These results also show that the agents were able to learn efficient rescue action because the reward distribution reflected contribution degree.

5. Conclusion

In this chapter, we considered rescue robots as a multi-agent system and proposed three reward distributions for the agents to learn cooperative action with consideration given to the condition of the injured and obstacle removal in responding to our disaster rescue problem, as well as investigating the timing of reward conferral on the agents.

Comparative experiments showed that the timing of reward distribution enabling the agents to obtain the most efficient cooperative actions consisted of reward conferral at the stages in which the agent discovered the injured person or obstacle and at completion of their transport. The results also showed that the capability of cooperative actions for the most efficient injured rescue and obstacle removal could be acquired through reward distribution by contribution degree in accordance with condition.

In this chapter, the multi-agent system corresponding to the disaster rescue problem, rescue simulations were performed with the condition of the injured determined in advance. In future studies, we plan to conduct simulations with dynamic changes over time in both the condition of the injured and removable versus nonremovable states of the obstacles.

Acknowledgements

This research was supported by the Japan Society for the Promotion of Science (JSPS) KAKENHI Grant Number JP16K01303.

Author details

Mengchun Xie
Department of Electrical and Computer Engineering, National Institute of Technology, Wakayama College, Wakayama-ken, Japan

*Address all correspondence to: xie@wakayama-nct.ac.jp

References

[1] Gautschi O, Cadosch D, Rajan G, Zellweger R. Earthquakes and trauma: Review of triage and injury-specific, immediate care. Prehospital and Disaster Medicine: The Official Journal of the National Association of EMS Physicians and the World Association for Emergency and Disaster Medicine in Association with the Acute Care Foundation. 2008;**23**(2):195-201. DOI: 10.1017/S1049023X00005847

[2] Xie M. Cooperative behavior rule acquisition for multi-agent systems by machine learning. In: Advances in Reinforcement Learning. Rijeka, Croatia: Intech; 2011. pp. 81-98

[3] Geron A. Hands-on Machine Learning with Scikit-Learn & TensorFlow. Sebastopol CA: O'Reilly Media Inc; 2018

[4] Sutton RS, Barto AG. Reinforcement Learning: An Introduction. Cambridge, Massachusetts, London, England: The MIT Press; 1998

[5] Conradie AVE, Aldrich C. Development of neurocontrollers with evolutionary reinforcement learning. Computers & Chemical Engineering. 2005;**30**:1-17

[6] Isbell CL, Shelton CR, Kearns M, Singh S, Stone P. A social reinforcement learning agent. In: Proceedings of the Fifth International Conference on Autonomous Agents. 2001. pp. 377-384

[7] Tatomir B, Rothkrantz L, Popa M. Intelligent system for exploring dynamic crisis environments. In: Proceeding of the Third International Conference on Information Systems for Crisis Response and Management. 2006

[8] Stone P, Veloso M. Using machine learning in the soccer server. In: Proc. of IROS-96 Workshop on Robocup. 1996

[9] Buford JF, Jakobson G, Lewis L. Multi-agent situation management for supporting large-scale disaster relief operations. The International Journal of Intelligent Control and Systems. 2006;**11**(4):284-295

[10] Matsubara H, Frank I, Tanaka K, et al. Automatic soccer commentary and RoboCup. In: The 2nd Proceedings of RoboCap Workshop. 1998

[11] Pereira R d P, Engel PM. A Framework for Constrained and Adaptive Behavior-Based Agents, arXiv preprint arXiv:1506.02312v12015. pp. 1-16

[12] Spychalski P, Arendt R. Machine learning in multi-agent systems using associative arrays. Parallel Computing. 2018;**75**:88-99

[13] Zhou P, Shen H. Multi-agent cooperation by reinforcement learning with teammate modeling and reward allotment. In: 8th International Conference on Fuzzy Systems and Knowledge Discovery; 4 February, 2011; FSKD. 2011. pp. 1316-1319

[14] Zemzemb W, Tagina M. Cooperative multi-agent systems using distributed reinforcement learning techniques. Procedia Computer Science. 2018;**126**:517-526

[15] Xie M, Murata M, Muraki Y. Tsunami evacuation guidance simulation using multi-agent systems based on OpenStreetMap. International Journal of Environmental Sciences. 2017;**2**:231-237. ISSN: 2367-8941

[16] Xie M, Murata M, Sato S. Acquisition of cooperative action by rescue agents with distributed roles. In: Leu G et al., editors. Intelligent and Evolutionary Systems, Proceedings in Adaptation, Learning and Optimization. Vol. 8. AG: Springer

International Publishing; 2017. pp. 483-493

[17] Jennings N, Sycara K, Wooldridge M. A roadmap of agent research and development. Autonomous Agents and Multi-Agent Systems. 1998;**1**:7-38

[18] Xie M. Representation of the perceived environment and acquisition of behavior rule for multi-agent systems by Q-learning. In: Proceedings of the 4th International Conference on Autonomous Robots and Agents. 2009. pp. 453-457

[19] Xie M, Tachibana A. Cooperative behavior acquisition for multi-agent systems by Q-learning. In: Proceedings IEEE Symposium on Foundations of Computational Intelligence. 2007. pp. 424-428

[20] Weiss G. Multiagent Systems: A Modern Approach to Distributed Artificial Intelligence. Cambridge, Massachusetts, London, England: The MIT Press; 2000

[21] Panait L, Luke S. Cooperative multi-agent learning: The state of the art. Autonomous Agents and Multi-Agent Systems. 2005;**11**(3):387-434

[22] Son TC, Pontelli E, Nguyen N. Planning for Multiagent Using ASP-Prolog, Computational Logic in Multi-Agent Systems. New York, USA: Springer; 2010. pp. 1-19

[23] Xie M, Okazaki K. Application of multi-agent systems to disaster relief using Q-learning. In: Proceedings of the IASTED International Conference on Software Engineering and Applications. Calgary, Alberta, Canada: ACAT Press; 2008. pp. 143-147

Chapter 10

A Cooperative Game Using the P300 EEG-Based Brain-Computer Interface

Kaoru Sumi, Keigo Yabuki, Thomas James Tiam-Lee, Abdelkader Nasreddine Belkacem, Quentin Ferre, Shogo Hirai and Teruto Endo

Abstract

In this paper, we present a cooperative game, Brainio Bros 300, using a brain-computer interface (BCI). The game is cooperatively controlled by two people using P300-generating color discrimination. The two users advance through the game together, one as the "player" and the other as the "supporter" providing assistance. We assumed that players would be able-bodied, while supporters would include people with severe disabilities. Through experiments using human subjects, we evaluated the subjects' impressions of the game and its usefulness. The results of the impression evaluation showed that the subjects generally had good impressions, and there were many opinions that such cooperative games are interesting. We also discuss the possibilities of using the P300 BCI.

Keywords: P300, brain computer interface, EEG, cooperative game, game for people with major disabilities, game design

1. Introduction

A brain-computer interface (BCI) offers a noninvasive means of enabling a human to send messages and commands directly from his or her brain to a computer without moving, by wearing a simple scalp probe (a set of electrodes or sensors) [1–4]. This noninvasive technology differs from invasive, surgical approaches that can cause irreversible damage to brain tissue.

In this paper, we present a BCI-based cooperative game, Brainio Bros 300. The BCI uses the P300 brain wave [5–9], a typical electrophysiological response to internal and external event-related potential (ERP) stimuli, measured using an EEG. The P300 wave has proven relatively easy to use for a variety of control-signaling purposes in much recent practical research.

When a human experiences interest in any kind of target, there is a measurable brain activity response. It is known that when a subject recognizes a specified photograph among a series of randomly presented photographs (i.e., the "ah!" response), P300 can be measured around the top of the head. Regardless of the type of stimulus (visual, tactile, auditory, olfactory, gustatory, etc.), P300 appears around 300 ms after the stimulus, which makes it a very useful brain feature that can be used by healthy or handicapped people for controlling an external device or communicating with the environment in real time. Notable applications of a P300 BCI include previous engineering studies in which a locomotive robot [10] and wheelchair [11] were controlled. Some neuroscientific experimental studies have also been conducted using "brain painting" [12, 13] for patient rehabilitation. A P300 BCI has also been used with virtual reality spaces [14] and as an interface for Twitter and Second Life [15].

Simple BCI games can also be useful for helping a user to control his or her brain activity. Games controlled using EEG signals have been designed to improve the power and duration of concentration, increase the speed and accuracy of brain waves, and improve cognitive function [16]. BCI-based games appear in both medical- and entertainment-focused varieties. Medical applications include games that use a steady-state visual evoked potential (SSVEP) to improve the concentration power necessary to control a BCI [17]. Here, SSVEPs refer to the brain signals induced by using a pattern reversal stimulus (i.e., the use of a checkerboard pattern to stimulate vision) or a flash stimulus (i.e., the use of a flickering light source such as an LED to stimulate vision). Medical games to promote the speedy generation of BCI commands, thus improving the user experience, have also been developed [18]. In the entertainment realm, games have been developed using a number of signals, including P300, to play popular games such as Pong and Tetris and to control a dancing robot [19–22]. Most such games depend on the player's degree of concentration [22].

In this research, we developed Brainio Bros 300 as a game controlled cooperatively by two people using P300-generating color discrimination. The two users advance together through the game, one as the "player" and the other as the "supporter" providing assistance. The player controls the game character by using a keyboard's arrow keys to navigate through a series of colored blocks, while the supporter removes blocks obstructing the player's path by thinking of the appropriate color via the P300 BCI. By cooperating, the participants can reach the end of the game. We assumed that players would be able-bodied, while supporters could include people with severe disabilities.

2. Brainio Bros 300 cooperative game

This section describes the Brainio Bros 300 game, with the discussion divided into two parts: the P300 BCI used and the components and design of the cooperative game.

2.1 P300-based brain-computer interface

We used a new, portable wireless EEG cap called g.Unicorn EEG (g.tec medical engineering, Austria), as shown in **Figure 1**, for recording brain activity in real time. For our experimental paradigm, we adapted the P300 speller idea to our problem by using MATLAB/Simulink to develop the game-based BCI. Ten dry electrodes were used to record EEG signals at a sampling frequency of 256 Hz. The electrodes were placed according to the international 10–20 system, using the Fz (forehead), Cz (crown), P3, Pz, P4, PO7, Oz, and PO8 (all at the back of the head) locations, with references placed at A2 (earlobe) and Fz (forehead), as shown in **Figure 2**.

Before the cooperative game begins, the first user (designated as the "supporter") had to put on the EEG cap and perform calibration for sending color commands. We developed a program enabling the user to calibrate six colors: red,

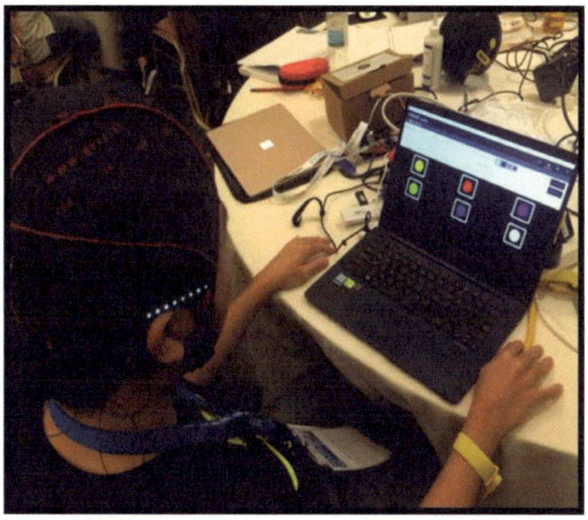

Figure 1.
Calibration of the EEG experiment using the g.Unicorn EEG cap for a P300-based BCI.

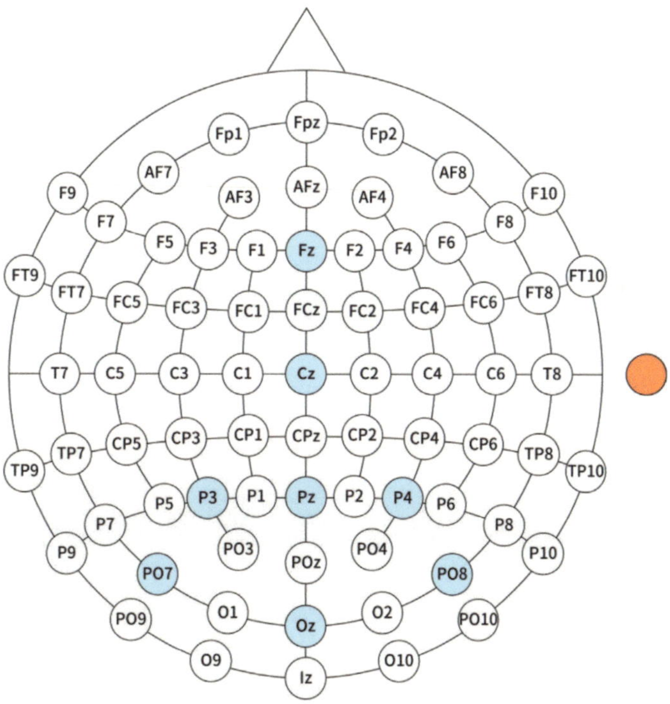

Figure 2.
Electrode positions of the eight channels.

blue, green, yellow, purple, and white. The six colors were randomly arranged into two rows of three, with each box flickering 30 times between a photograph of a human face and a color. The subject choses a color and counted in their head how many times that color was displayed. Because research results have indicated that flickering photographs of famous people increases calibration accuracy by increasing the amplitude of the P300 wave, we used images of widely recognizable people, such as Albert Einstein and President Donald Trump. The procedures of the calibration and game phases are detailed below:

- Calibration phase

  1. Select the colors to be used in calibration, as illustrated in **Figure 3**. For example, red, blue, green, and yellow can be displayed in order, as shown in the figure under "Item selections."
  2. Begin calibration.
  3. The system directs the user to look at "red."
  4. The colors randomly flicker. The user mentally adds to the count every time he or she sees the color red. After red has flickered 30 times, the system is configured to stop.
  5. The system records the speed of the response every time the color red was flashed and the EEG information.
  6. This process continues three–five more times for all the other colors. Each color takes 20 s, for a total of around 2 min.

- Game phase

  1. As colors are randomly flashed on the screen, the user looks at the color he or she wants to select and mentally counts its flashes. We used 20 flashes for a balance between selection accuracy and enjoyability of the game.
  2. The system guesses which color the user selected according to how the EEG changes. The EEG readings at these moments are measured, and the instants at which the low-frequency stimuli are displayed are averaged as the trigger.

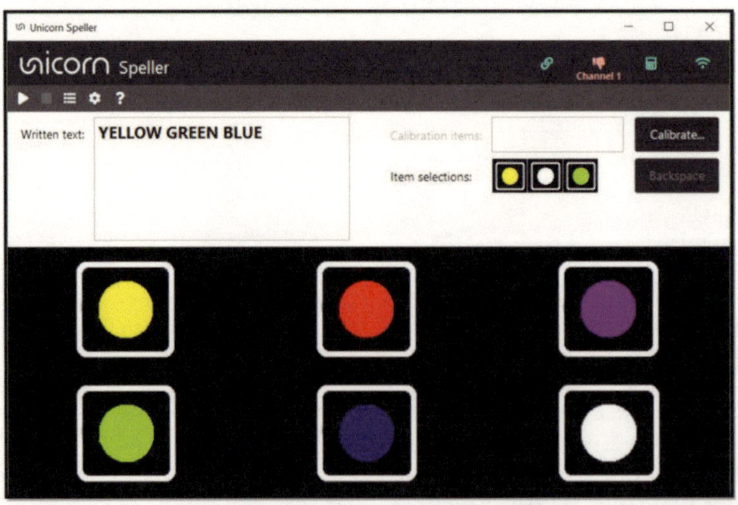

Figure 3.
Calibration screen for our P300 experimental paradigm.

The information on the selected color was sent by a UDP broadcast on port 1000 and received by a Unity application. As seen in **Figure 3**, the selected colors were also shown under "Written text," but this was not actually used in the game.

2.2 Brainio Bros 300 design

The Brainio Bros 300 cooperative game was developed in Unity 2018 and runs on the Windows 10 operating system. It is a game in the style of Nintendo's Super Mario Bros., in which the player maneuvers a character through various obstacles to reach a goal flag and complete the stage. Along the way, the player encounters blocks that are too high to clear and points where it is impossible to pass, but the player and supporter work together to complete the game.

The game contains blocks of five colors: red, blue, green, yellow, and purple. **Figure 4** illustrates a green block obstructing the player, preventing him or her from advancing. In such situation, the player communicates an instruction to the supporter (e.g., "green's in the way" or "destroy green"), and the supporter then thinks of the color green. By doing so, the green block in the game can be destroyed, as shown in **Figure 5**. The game was designed so that it cannot be completed without the player and supporter cooperating.

Because the game would not be enjoyable with only one obstruction, multiple blocks of different colors are placed in one spot, as shown in **Figure 4**, requiring the player to consider which color to destroy. The game was also designed to offer multiple courses, allowing the player to choose his or her own course. For example, **Figure 6** shows a case of two paths. If the red block is destroyed, the player can

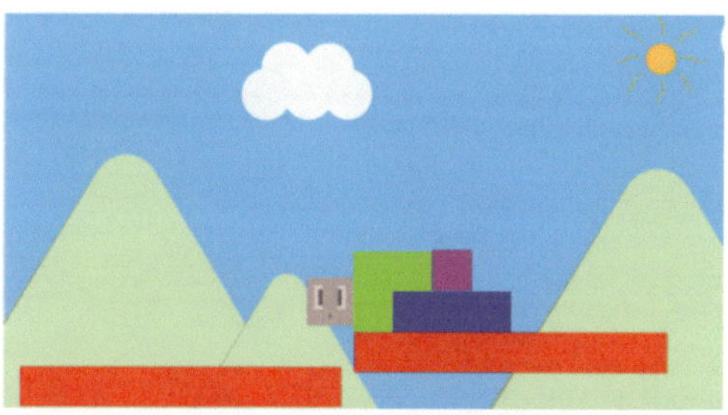

Figure 4.
Obstructed by the green block.

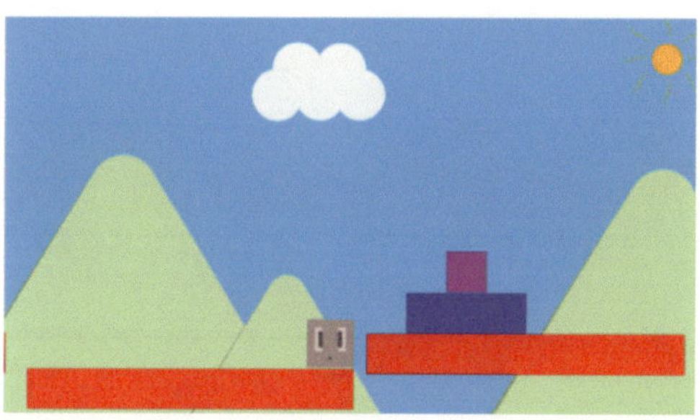

Figure 5.
After destroying the green block.

advance via the blue block, whereas if the blue block is destroyed, the player can jump onto the red block and continue onward.

The game was designed to destroy (i.e., hide) only the one color currently recognized by the BCI, so that only one color could be destroyed at a time. For example, if a red block is first destroyed and then a green block, the game displays the destroyed red block again. **Figure 7** shows a case of the player unable to advance with only a blue block displayed, while **Figure 8** shows the result with the blue block destroyed, causing the red blocks to reappear. The game was designed as indicated by these images, so that, even though there are no blocks beyond the blue block, destroying the blue block causes the red blocks to reappear, allowing the player to advance.

This system, with the combined limitations of using only five colors and allowing only one color to be destroyed at a time, gives the player manual control over which blocks are destroyed. Because an unintended color can be destroyed, it is

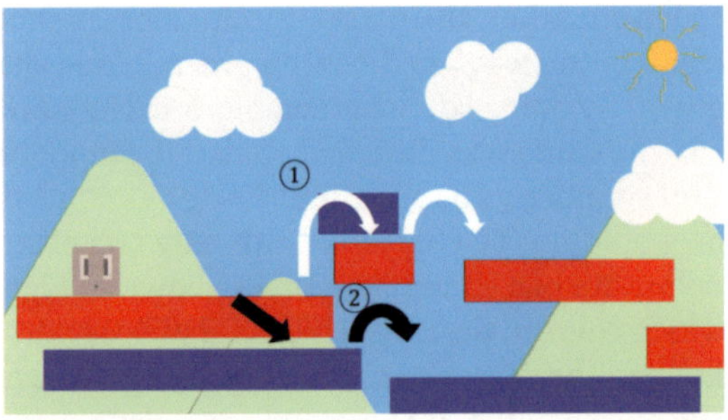

Figure 6.
Start screen with two ways of advancing.

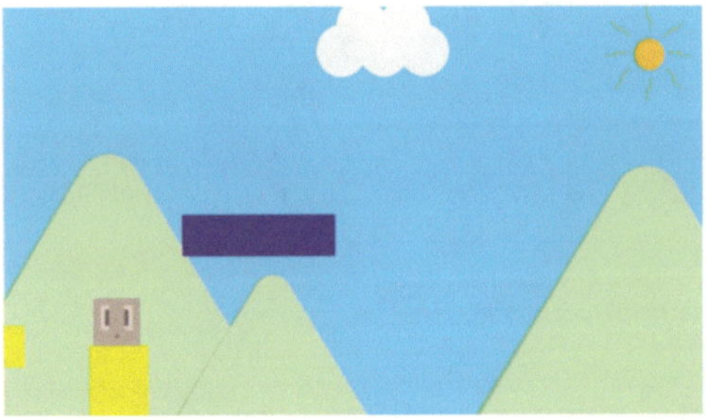

Figure 7.
Unable to reach the blue block.

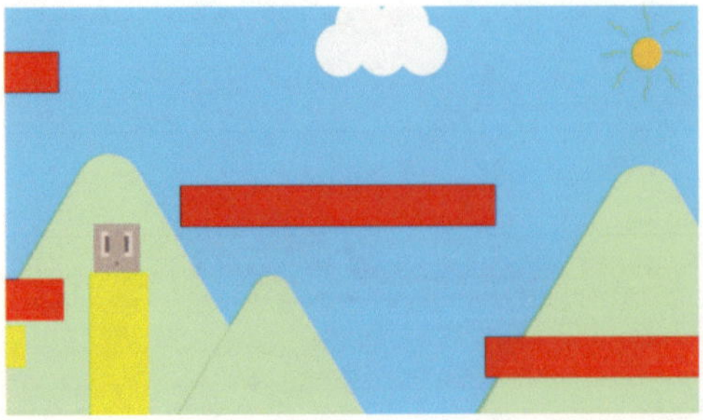

Figure 8.
Blue block destroyed, causing red blocks to reappear.

possible to destroy the player character's foothold. When the character falls, however, it returns to the start point, from where the player can continue the game.

The game also features obstacles in which blocks move horizontally or vertically. Such blocks were programmed in advance to behave as such in the game in advance. We included such features to prevent the game from becoming a monotonous experience for the users. A flag is beyond all the obstacles. When the character touches the flag, the game is completed.

3. Game experiment

For experiments using an EEG capable of measuring the P300 brain wave, it is extremely difficult at present to prepare an environment supporting easy calibration for many subjects. For example, even preparing only one EEG device capable of measuring P300 requires a considerable cost, and it takes time to perform the calibration. Therefore, this paper considers the possibilities of games for use with such a BCI by focusing on evaluating the Brainio Bros 300 game.

Specifically, we evaluated Brainio Bros 300 in terms of the user's impression of the game and its usefulness. For our methodology, we used the Wizard of Oz (WOZ) approach. A WOZ system involves a user interacting with a person acting as a computer system (i.e., the "wizard"), allowing for effective simulation of a real system [23].

For Brainio Bros 300, although the supporter wore the EEG device, the game was actually controlled with a keyboard. We thus conducted an evaluation experiment with the supporter as a reference.

The experiment was conducted with 25 students at Future University Hakodate: 19 men and 6 women. Of these students, 12 were designated as supporters and 13 as players. The supporters consisted of 8 men and 4 women, while the players consisted of 11 men and 2 women. The average age of the whole group was 20.76 years, with average ages of 20.75 and 20.77 years for the supporter and player groups, respectively.

To use the WOZ approach, we created an experimental system using keyboard input to destroy blocks as a substitute for the P300 BCI component of Super Brainio Bros 300. In this system, pressing the "R," "G," "B," "Y," or "C" keys caused the red, green, blue, yellow, or purple blocks, respectively, to be destroyed. For the ease of distinguishing which key corresponded to which color, we applied a sticker of each color to its corresponding key.

We also created a post-experiment questionnaire to evaluate the users' impressions and opinions of the usefulness of Super Brainio Bros 300. **Table 1** lists the details of the questionnaire, which included questions using the semantic differential (SD) method, a five-point scale method, and free responses. For the five-point scale, the responses consisted of "strongly agree," "agree," "neither," "disagree," and "strongly disagree." The questions are listed with abbreviated forms in the table.

Table 2 lists the details of each condition for the SD method and the reasons for its selection. Each condition showing a positive impression is filled in gray. On the questionnaire form, the positive and negative responses were distributed between the left and right sides as a counterbalancing measure. The SD method used a seven-stage evaluation, with responses consisting of "extremely" (positive or negative), "very" (positive or negative), "a little" (positive or negative), and "neither."

We also used a keyboard, display, notebook PC, desk, chair, and EEG headset as experimental materials, arranged as shown in **Figure 9**.

Question (abbreviated)	Question form	Question text (full)
SD Method	SD Method	Please circle the adjective which most accurately reflects the intuitive impression you received from using the system. Please do not think too deeply, but answer based on your first impression.
Was it interesting?	5-point method	Was this game interesting (fun, enjoyable)? Please circle the response that applies.
Reasons it was interesting	Free response	What aspects, specifically, did you find interesting (fun, enjoyable)?
Did you get along?	5-point method	Do you think you got along with the person you played together with? Please circle the response that applies.
Communicating with disabled person	5-point method	Do you think this game would be useful for communicating with a disabled person? Please circle the response that applies.
Communicating with a child	5-point method	Do you think this game would be useful for communicating with a child? Please circle the response that applies.
Other future uses	Free response	How else do you think this game could be used in future?
Did you want to keep playing?	5-point method	If the game kept going, would you want to keep playing it? Please circle the response that applies.
Game design	5-point method	Was the game screen easy to understand? Please circle the response that applies.
Would you recommend it?	5-point method	Would you recommend this game to others (friends, family etc.)? Please circle the response that applies.
Points for improvement	Free response	What feature, functions etc. would make you more likely to recommend this game to others?
Other opinions and thoughts	Free response	If you have any other thoughts or opinions about this system, please note them here.

Table 1.
Questionnaire details.

We next describe the experimental procedure. The total experiment time was around 30 minutes. The first step was to gather all the subjects in a room and form them into pairs. The participants were instructed to pair with someone they did not know, where possible. As there was an odd number of participants, resulting in one excess player, a researcher acted as the supporter for that player and did not fill out a questionnaire. After pairing the participants, we explained the experiment to the whole group. This included explanations of the following: (1) an overview of the game (a game controlled by brain waves, requiring the player and supporter to cooperate to reach the goal), (2) the role of the player (to control the character by using the keyboard), (3) the role of the supporter (to assist the player by using brain waves), (4) the control method, and (5) an image of the game screen. The players were then taken into separate rooms containing the experimental materials. Each player was seated in the chair indicated by "Player's chair" in **Figure 9** and asked to wait until the supporter arrived.

Condition		Reason for selection
Positive impression	Negative impression	
Satisfying	Unsatisfying	Game's level of satisfaction
Full	Dull	Game's fullness
Cooperative	Uncooperative	Quality of the pair's cooperative play
Enjoyable	Unenjoyable	Favorability towards the game
Happy	Sad	Change in feelings due to the game
Simple	Complex	Nature of the entire game
Cute	Ugly	Appeal of the game design
Creative	Cliché	Game's creativity
New	Old	Game's novelty
Cool	Uncool	Game's creativity (2)
Friendly	Distant	Impression of game
Easy	Difficult	Game's difficulty
Lively	Gloomy	Game's fullness (2)
Rich	Empty	Game's creativity
Varied	Monotonous	Awareness of changing features

Table 2.
Details of the conditions used for the SD method, together with the reasons for their use.

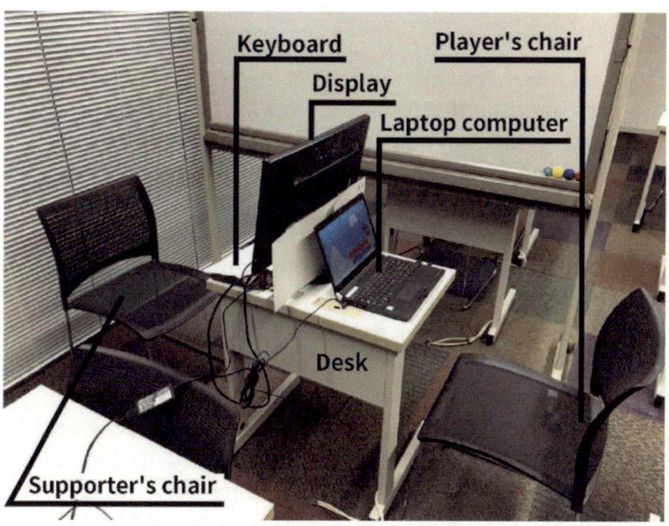

Figure 9.
Arrangement of the experimental materials.

After the players had been moved, we explained to the supporters that this experiment used the WOZ approach, that brain waves were not actually used, and that they would advance through the game by using the keyboard. The supporters were asked to wear the EEG headset and appear to the player as if they were controlling the game through brain waves. The supporters were then taken to the separate rooms in which the players were waiting, and each was seated in the "Supporter's chair" shown in **Figure 9**. As soon as we had confirmed that the player and supporter were both seated, a brief explanation was once again provided to both of them. At this time, the participants were instructed to communicate regarding the color of the block when the player wanted a certain block cleared, when the supporter was trying to clear a block, and so on.

After this instruction, the participants began playing the game. After they had completed it, they returned to the room where the initial explanation had been provided, and they filled out the questionnaires. Once they had completed the questionnaires, the experiment was over. At this point, they were instructed not to reveal the details of the experiment.

Finally, we explain our analysis methods for the experimental data. For the SD method in which pairs of words were displayed side by side (e.g., easy vs. difficult) to assess the impression of the participants, they were asked to assign a score in the range of −3 and 3, with 0 representing "neither", −3 representing "extremely leaning to the left word", and 3 representing "extremely leaning to the right word". We then compiled descriptive statistics and plotted a semantic profile.

Next, the five-point scale was tallied with "strongly agree" as 5 points, "agree" as 4 points, "neither" as 3 points, "disagree" as 2 points, and "strongly disagree" as 1 point. After compiling descriptive statistics for this data, we performed a chi-square test.

Finally, for the free responses, we counted experiences and keywords shared among participants and collected them into overall viewpoints. We also collected strongly held minority opinions as necessary.

4. Results

Table 3 and **Figure 10** give the results of the SD method. **Table 3** lists the average for each question for each participant role, as well as the difference between the groups. The fields shown in gray indicate a response that implies a positive impression. The left/right distribution of the response fields is the same as on the questionnaire sheet provided to the participants. Averages and average differences with an absolute value greater than 1 are also shown in gray. We also conducted semantic profiling based on the results, as shown in **Figure 10**.

From the group differences indicated by this table and graph, we observed no great differences between the impressions of the supporters and players. The average values in gray show that "substantial," "cooperative," "enjoyable," "happy," "cute," "friendly," and "lively" were evaluated highly by both players and supporters, with "cooperative" evaluated particularly highly. Moreover, the players highly evaluated "satisfying" and "new."

Because all the data fell within one standard deviation, we could conclude that it was a good set of low-variance data. In the grayed averages, we also see that both supporters and players rated "Was it interesting?" and "Interacting with a child" highly. Players alone rated "Game design" and "Would recommend" highly.

Table 4 and **Figure 11** show the five-point scale responses, organized by the participants' roles, in terms of averages and standard deviations (**Table 4**) and percentages (**Figure 11**). **Table 4** shows averages greater than 4 in gray. In addition,

Condition		Supporter	Player	Difference between groups
Left response	Right response			
Satisfying	Unsatisfying	-0.67	-1.31	0.64
Dull	Full	1.00	1.38	-0.38
Cooperative	Uncooperative	-2.00	-2.08	0.08
Enjoyable	Unenjoyable	-1.17	-1.62	0.45
Sad	Happy	1.25	1.15	0.10
Complex	Simple	0.42	0.08	0.34
Ugly	Cute	1.00	1.00	0.00
Creative	Cliché	-0.67	-0.85	0.18
New	Old	-0.83	-1.00	0.17
Cool	Uncool	-0.75	-0.92	0.17
Distant	Friendly	1.42	1.08	0.34
Difficult	Easy	0.17	-0.08	0.24
Lively	Gloomy	-1.00	-1.08	0.08
Empty	Rich	0.33	0.85	-0.51
Varied	Monotonous	-0.42	-0.77	0.35

Table 3.
SD method results.

Table 5 lists the sums of the percentages of "strongly agree" and "agree" responses to each question, as well as the results of the chi-square test. The percentages in gray indicate values above 80%, while the statistical significances in gray indicate a significant statistic at the 5% significance level. The analysis shows that "Would you recommend it?" had a significant result at the 5% level, while the results of the remaining six questions were significant at a significance level of 10%.

Finally, we will discuss the participants' free responses, including particularly common responses and useful minority opinions. First, out of the people who responded that "it was interesting", 9 out of the 12 supporters and 8 out of the 13 players gave "cooperative play" as a reason.

For "Other future uses," 6 out of 12 supporters offered "use as an icebreaker" as a response, as did 4 out of 13 players. In addition, notable minority opinions

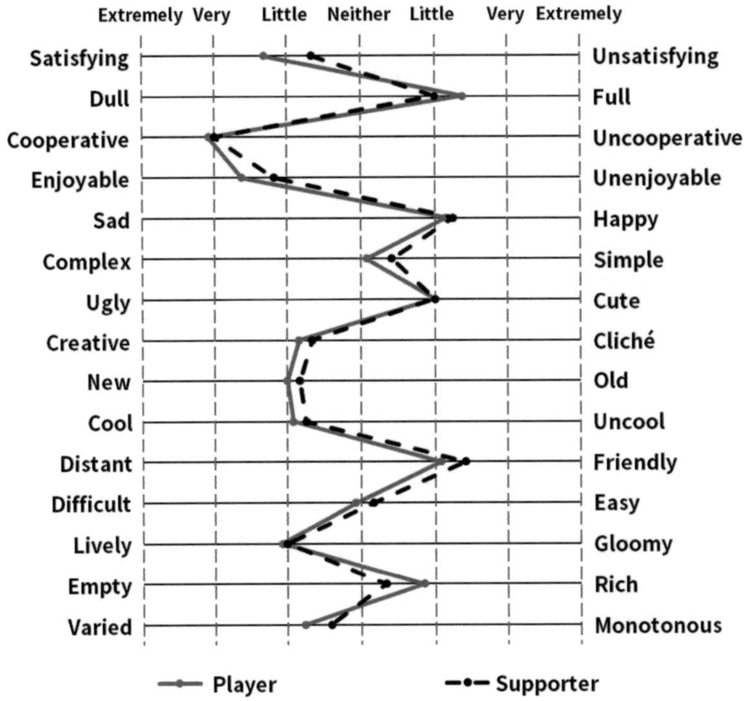

Figure 10.
Semantic profile of the SD method.

Question (abbreviated)	Supporter		Player	
	Average value	SD	Average value	SD
Was it interesting?	4.00	0.85	4.23	0.60
Did you get along?	3.67	0.65	3.62	0.77
Communicating with disabled person	3.25	0.75	3.77	0.60
Communicating with a child	4.17	0.39	4.23	0.60
Did you want to keep playing?	3.67	0.98	3.92	0.86
Game design	3.75	0.75	4.23	0.60
Would you recommend it?	3.00	0.95	4.15	0.38

Table 4.
Averages and standard deviations for the five-point scale method.

included "use in brain training," "communication with foreigners," and "prevention of dementia in the elderly."

As for "Points for improvement," 2 out of 12 supporters mentioned the addition of more complex features and the ability to actually play using brain waves. Of the 13 players, 2 mentioned the ability to use items and the appearance of enemies in the game as points for improvement. Additionally, one minority opinion suggested the capability of the player, too, to use brain waves to control the game.

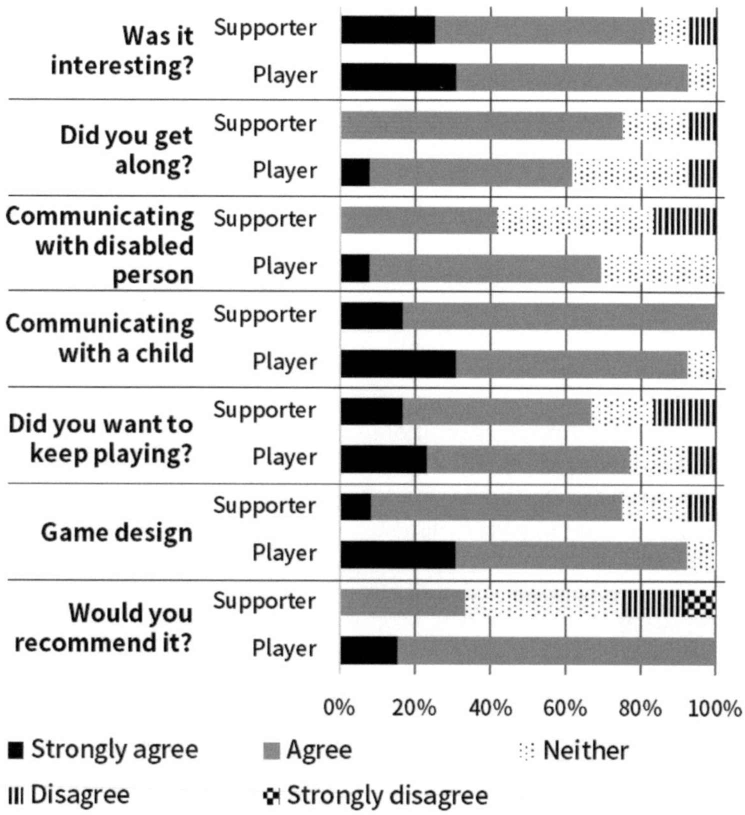

Figure 11.
Percentage results for the five-point scale method.

Question (abbreviated)	Percentage of "Strongly believe" and "Believe"	χ^2	df	Sig.
Was it interesting?	92.3%	5.69	2	p<.1
Did you get along?	61.5%	7.62	3	p<.1
Communicating with disabled person	69.2%	5.69	2	p<.1
Communicating with a child	92.3%	5.69	2	p<.1
Did you want to keep playing?	76.9%	6.39	3	p<.1
Game design	92.3%	5.69	2	p<.1
Would you recommend it?	100%	6.23	1	p<.05

Table 5.
Percentage sums of the players' "strongly agree" and "agree" responses and chi-square test results.

Finally, for "Any other opinions or feelings," many supporters and players mentioned that the game was interesting and fun.

5. Discussion

We conducted an impression evaluation of the Brainio Bros 300 cooperative game and its usefulness. First, the results of the SD method showed that the players evaluated the game as "full," "cooperative," "enjoyable," "happy," "cute," "friendly," "lively," "satisfying," and "new," with "cooperative" evaluated particularly highly. On the five-point scale, the game was evaluated highly in terms of both the players' average values and the combined percentages of "strongly agree" and "agree" for the questions of "Interesting," "Communicating with a child," "Game design," and "Would recommend," with "Would recommend" showing a particularly strong correlation. Finally, the opinion that the cooperative aspect of play was interesting was particularly widely expressed in the free responses.

One of the biggest advantages of Brainio Bros 300 is the capability for the player, who does not have to wear an EEG cap, to play together with the supporter, who does wear an EEG cap. We believe that playing cooperative games using a P300 BCI could be of significant benefit to people with major disabilities such as amyotrophic lateral sclerosis (ALS), enabling them to play with able-bodied children, family members, and friends, thus deepening connections and communication.

The use of a P300 BCI is an easy-to-measure, noninvasive method. It can also be controlled with a high degree of accuracy without the need for detailed user training in advance. Training the P300 BCI command categories does not take a great deal of time. Most patients, including almost all able-bodied people and even people with severe paralysis, can use a P300 BCI. It also offers a goal-oriented control signal that is particularly suited to situations that do not require a continuous control signal.

On the other hand, one of the game's limitations is as follows. The P300 BCI is one of the fastest of the currently usable BCIs, but it is still very slow compared to normal input devices such as mice and game controllers. In the current Brainio Bros 300 system, the player must wait for the colors to flash before having the supporter select a color.

With the development of a decoding algorithm that could detect the P300 brain wave to a high degree of accuracy after only one attempt, a command could be sent to the game every second. The results could then be adjusted according to feedback following categorization. For example, in the event of a mistaken command, the response time could be minimized by testing the supporter again. This should also allow the result to be checked once per second. Although Brainio Bros P300 is a game in which players and supporters cooperate, it takes time for a supporter to erase blocks by using P300 control as compared to standard games. Moreover, as it is a game in which two people cooperate, it differs from a competitive game based on speed. For this reason, a player and a supporter must play together and possibly become friends.

We believe that, in the future, if it is possible to reduce the number of flashes while maintaining the current level of accuracy and to increase the number of commands (controllable dimensions), this type of game would be usable in the real world and present an extremely promising interface.

Some problems with using a P300 BCI are that real-time P300 detection can sometimes be inaccurate, as it is easily affected by a number of human sensory phenomena such as attentional blinking, repetition blindness, and change blindness [24–28]. It is also possible for motivation to impact BCI performance [29], causing the EEG signal pattern to change according to the attention level, fatigue, state of mind, learning, and unsteadiness [1]. A P300 BCI might also not be an effective method for people who cannot control their line of sight [30]. It is thus important to work carefully, given the potential impacts of participants' state of mind and attention to the problem.

6. Conclusion

In this BCI-based game research, we developed a real-time game, Brainio Bros 300, a cooperative game using a P300 BCI to facilitate two users (a player, who controls the character in the game and does not wear an EEG cap, and a supporter, who uses his or her brain activity to communicate) working together to achieve one goal. We evaluated participants' impressions of the game and its usefulness and considered the viability of the P300 BCI interface.

In the future, we would like to use noninvasive measurement to investigate more deeply the brain mechanism during a cooperative video game.

Acknowledgements

This research was a first place winner, IEEE Brain Winner, and BR41N.IO SfN Winner at the IEEE SMC2018 BCI Hackathon. On receipt of these awards, we would like to express our gratitude to g.tec and to all the organizers, as well as all the students, who assisted with our experiment.

Author details

Kaoru Sumi[1*], Keigo Yabuki[1], Thomas James Tiam-Lee[1], Abdelkader Nasreddine Belkacem[2,3], Quentin Ferre[4], Shogo Hirai[1] and Teruto Endo[5]

1 Future University Hakodate, Hakodate, Japan

2 Osaka University, Osaka, Japan

3 United Arab Emirates University, Al Ain, UAE

4 Universite Paris-Est Marne-la-Vallee, Paris, France

5 Tohoku Institute of Technology, Sendai, Japan

*Address all correspondence to: kaoru.sumi@acm.org

References

[1] Wolpaw J, Birbaumer N, McFarland D, Pfurtscheller G, Vaughan T. Brain-computer interfaces for communication and control. Clinical Neurophysiology. 2002;**113**:767-791

[2] Krucoff MO, Rahimpour S, Slutzky MW, Edgerton VR, Turner DA. Enhancing nervous system recovery through neurobiologics, neural interface training, and neurorehabilitation. Neuroprosthetics. 2016;**10**:584. DOI: 10.3389/fnins.2016.00584. PMC 5186786. PMID 28082858

[3] Vidal JJ. Toward direct brain-computer communication. Annual Review of Biophysics and Bioengineering. 1973;**2**(1):157-180. DOI: 10.1146/annurev.bb.02.060173.001105. PMID 4583653

[4] Vidal J. Real-time detection of brain events in EEG. IEEE Proceedings. 1977; **65**(5):633-641. DOI: 10.1109/PROC.1977.10542

[5] Piccione F, Giorgi F, Tonin P, et al. P300-based brain computer interface: Reliability and performance in healthy and paralysed participants. Clinical Neurophysiology. 2006;**117**(3):531-537. DOI: 10.1016/j.clinph.2005.07.024. PMID 16458069

[6] Donchin E, Spencer KM, Wijesinghe R. The mental prosthesis: Assessing the speed of a P300-based brain–computer interface. IEEE Transactions on Rehabilitation Engineering. 2000;**8**(2):174-179. DOI: 10.1109/86.847808

[7] Nijboer F, Sellers EW, Mellinger J, et al. A P300-based brain–computer interface for people with amyotrophic lateral sclerosis. Clinical Neurophysiology. 2008;**119**:1909-1916. DOI: 10.1016/j.clinph.2008.03.034. PMC 2853977. PMID 18571984

[8] Sutton S, Tueting P, Zubin J, John E. Information delivery and the sensory evoked potential. Science. 1967;**155**: 1436-1439

[9] Farwell L, Donchin E. Talking off the top of your head: Toward a mental prosthesis utilizing event-related brain potentials. Electroencephalography and Clinical Neurophysiology. 1988;**70**: 510-523

[10] Bell CJ, Shenoy P, Chalodhorn R, Rao RPN. Control of a humanoid robot by a noninvasive brain-computer interface in humans. Journal of Neural Engineering. 2008;**5**:214

[11] Iturrate I, Antelis JM, Kubler A, Minguez J. A noninvasive brain-actuated wheelchair based on a P300 neurophysiological protocol and automated navigation. IEEE Education Society. 2009;**25**:614-627

[12] Kübler A, Halder S, Furdea A, Hösle A. Brain painting—BCI meets art. In: Proceedings of the 4th International Brain-Computer Interface Workshop and Training Course. Graz: University of Graz; 2008. pp. 361-366

[13] Muenssinger JI, Halder S, Kleih SC, Furdea A, Raco V, Hoesle A, et al. Frontiers: Brain painting: First evaluation of a new brain-computer interface application with ALS-patients and healthy volunteers. Frontiers in Neuroscience. 2010;**4**. DOI: 10.3389/fnins.2010.00182

[14] Edlinger G, Holzner C, Groenegress C, Guger C, Slater M. Goal-oriented control with brain-computer interface. Found. Augmented Cogn. Neuroergon. Oper. Neurosci. **5638**:732-740

[15] Edlinger G, Guger C. Social environments, mixed communication and goal-oriented control application

using a brain-computer interface. Universal Access in Human-Computer Interaction. Users Diversity. 2011;**6766**: 545-554

[16] Wolpaw JR, Wolpaw EW. Brain-Computer Interface: Principles and Practice. 1st ed. New York, NY, USA: Oxford University Press; 2012

[17] Lalor EC, Kelly SP, Finucane C, et al. Steady-state VEP-based brain-computer interface control in an immersive 3D gaming environment. Eurasip Journal on Applied Signal Processing. 2005, 2005;(19):3156-3164

[18] Marshall D, Coyle D, Wilson S, Callaghan M. Games, gameplay, and BCI: The state of the art. IEEE Transactions on Computational Intelligence and AI in Games. 2013;**5**(2): 82-99

[19] Finke A, Lenhardt A, Ritter H. The mindgame: A P300-based brain-computer interface game. Neural Networks. 2009;**22**(9):1329-1333

[20] Tangermann M, Krauledat M, Grzeska K, et al. Playing pinball with non-invasive BCI. Advances in Neural Information Processing Systems. 2009; **21**:1641-1648

[21] Wang Q, Sourina O, Nguyen MK. Fractal dimension based neurofeedback in serious games. The Visual Computer. 2011;**27**(4):299-309

[22] Kaufmann T, Schulz S, Grünzinger C, Kübler A. Flashing characters with famous faces improves ERP-based brain-computer interface performance. Journal of Neural Engineering. 2011;**8**: 056016. DOI: 10.1088/1741-2560/8/5/056016

[23] Bella M, Hanington B. Universal Methods of Design. Beverly, MA: Rockport Publishers; 2012. p. 204

[24] Fazel-Rezai R. Human error in P300 speller paradigm for brain-computer interface. In: The 29th Annual International Conference of the IEEE Engineering in Medicine and Biology Society. Lyon: IEEE EMBS; 2007. pp. 2516-2519

[25] Fazel-Rezai R. P300-based speller brain-computer interface. In: Naik GR, editor. Recent Advances in Biomedical Engineering. Austria: IN-TECH; 2009. pp. 137-148

[26] Citi L, Poli R, Cinel C, Sepulveda F. P300-based BCI mouse with genetically-optimized analogue control. IEEE Transactions on Neural Systems and Rehabilitation Engineering. 2008; **16**:51-61

[27] Jin J, Horki P, Brunner C, Wang X, Neuper C, Pfurtscheller G. A new P300 stimulus presentation pattern for EEG-based spelling systems. Biomedizinische Technik. Biomedical Engineering. 2010; **55**:203-210

[28] Townsend G, Lapallo B, Boulay C, Krusienski D, Frye G, Hauser C, et al. A novel P300-based brain-computer interface stimulus presentation paradigm: Moving beyond rows and columns. Clinical Neurophysiology. 2010;**121**:1109-1120

[29] Kleih S, Kaufmann T, Zickler C, Halder S, Leotta F, Cincotti F, et al. Out of the frying pan into the fire—The P300 based BCI faces real world challenges. Progress in Brain Research. 2012;**194**:27-46

[30] Brunner P, Joshi S, Briskin S, Wolpaw J, Bischof H, Schalk G. Does the 'P300' speller depend on eye gaze? Journal of Neural Engineering. 2010;7: 056013